DO NOT REMOVE
CARDS FROM POCKET

Day Care Programs for Alzheimer's Disease and Related Disorders

Day Care Programs for Alzheimer's Disease and Related Disorders

John Panella, Jr., M.A., M.P.H.

Program Director
Darien Convalescent Center
Darien, Connecticut

Demos Publications • New York

Demos Publications, 156 Fifth Avenue, New York, New York 10010

Made in the United States of America

Library of Congress Cataloging in Publication Data

Main entry under title:
Day Care Programs for Alzheimer's Disease and Related Disorders
LC 87-71317
ISBN 0-939957-05-1

To Debbie
For your unwavering support

Acknowledgments

I would like to thank Dr. Fletcher H. McDowell, M.D., executive medical director of The Burke Rehabilitation Center, which I was affiliated with while this book was being written, for his constant encouragement. Without his assistance, I might never have met Dr. Diana M. Schneider of Demos Publications, whose support and technical guidance were neverending. A special and sincere note of thanks is due the present and former staff of the Dementia Day Care Program at The Burke Rehabilitation Center. Their creativity, special talents and keen perceptions of the patients' needs are visible throughout each chapter. Their willingness to "go the distance" is a virtue I greatly appreciate. I am also grateful to Maxine and Detria who painstakingly typed the first draft of this manuscript.

Preface

This book is addressed primarily to those individuals who presently are working in or planning a day care program for patients with Alzheimer's disease and related disorders. Its main goals are to share proven day care program ideas and strategies, and to encourage the refinement of programs that address the particular needs of individuals with these disorders.

Day care programs for patients with dementia have multiple goals, which include balancing the direct needs of the patient with the needs of their caregivers, the community, and the center itself. The relationships between the day care program staff, families, and patients are discussed in practical detail.

The range of sophistication of day care programs is enormous and no one formula for staffing, physical space design, or program planning can be universally applied. Readers therefore will not find any rigid sets of guidelines. Those individuals or groups that are developing new day care programs can use the information in this volume as a foundation for planning. Whenever appropriate, alternative approaches for varied day care settings are presented.

Each chapter highlights specific objectives and problem areas, emphasizing practical information that will be useful both to new and to existing centers. A wide range of topics is considered, including the development of physical facilities, staffing, admission and discharge policies, the development of activity programs, caregiver support programs, and financial management and recordkeeping.

A main theme throughout the book emphasizes how staff in day care programs can learn to structure the activities and environment to both help reduce behavior problems and to maximize the creative potential remaining in each patient. The reader is encouraged to examine the material and relate it to his or her own experience.

While the intended audience for this book is human service professionals, other specialists in education, private and governmental planning, and training will find it useful in providing an organized overview of day care for dementia.

Contents

Goals and Objectives of Day Care Programs for Patients with Alzheimer's Disease and Related Disorders

The principal goal of this book is to share proven program ideas and management techniques with those involved in the development, organization, and leadership of day care programs for patients with Alzheimer's disease and related disorders. While it emphasizes the experience of the Dementia Day Care Program at The Burke Rehabilitation Center, its purpose is not to replicate that model.

A more realistic objective is to encourage the funding and refinement of programs that address the particular needs of individuals with these disorders. Day care programs for those with dementia should not be considered a replacement for nursing homes or traditional day care for the elderly, and discussion concerning the development of programs specifically for the cognitively impaired are in no way meant to be adversarial to already existing institutions and centers that care for the elderly.

The development of a day care program for those with cognitive impairment requires extensive planning and development. Each chapter of this book highlights specific objectives and problem areas. Use the suggestions as a guide in formulating your own program. Each day care program will reflect the expertise and creativity of its staff, and each will develop a unique "mission."

The starting point for any day care program will be the development of the center's goals and objectives. A critical component is to develop goals for all those affected by the program—the patients themselves, their families and caregivers, and the day care center itself.

Caregivers

The true "consumers" of the day care program are the caregivers, not the patients, and it is through their actions that a prospective patient is evaluated and admitted to a program. A growing body of literature suggests that caregivers are better able to care for individuals with dementia when they are freed from the stress of daily care at regular intervals.

Goals for the caregiver include:

Respite time, scheduled time periods when the caregiver is not caring for the patient. Family members consistently report that they are better able to manage when they have such regularly scheduled respite periods. Day care programs allow families time that is theirs to use as they wish for a variety of private activities. The benefits of respite time do not necessarily require daily attendance. Two or three periods each week are sufficient to boost the caregiver's morale and make the time spent with the patient more pleasant.

Family assistance; through training, support and counseling, day programs can assist caregivers to better adapt to the continued decline of the patient. Educational and emotional support systems relieve the constant pressure involved in this stressful situation (see also chapter 10 on caregiver support systems).

The **development and communication of management techniques** allows families to learn and share specific approaches that can make daily living easier and more enjoyable. Issues are addressed such as home safety, wandering, and incontinence. Caregivers often feel less helpless when they have information and proven management techniques at their disposal, and families report satisfaction in becoming active participants in the care of their demented relative. Management skills must be learned; they are not innate.

Crisis intervention; the day program is often a "safety net" that provides support and referral to families facing crises associated with the care of their relative, such as the need for nursing home placement, violence in the home, and medication difficulties.

Patients

A very different set of goals exists for the patients, or group members, of the day program, which change as the patient becomes more cognitively impaired. Staff and family members take an increasingly active role in determining the patient's goals as his capacity for self-determination decreases. These may include:

A safe and supportive environment. Most patients, regardless of their level of cognitive impairment, will develop a sense of security in the day program. Staff members must clearly communicate to the patient that problems such as memory loss, aphasia, and incontinence can be managed and are not grounds for discharge. A day program that has been designed to meet the specific needs of the cognitively impaired individual will provide a safety net.

Role development. Chronic dementing illnesses slowly strip away people's "roles." Day programs reduce isolation and provide a specific place for the individual to socialize among his peers. Each patient develops a unique role in the day program; some think of it as a club or school, while others are aware enough to understand its real purpose. A good program will provide an atmosphere that blurs differences in backgrounds and economic status and allows patients to develop new roles with which they can adequately cope.

The program **fosters group spirit.** Despite cognitive and behavioral impairment, an individual's capacity to enjoy a wide range of emotions and experiences does not end with the diagnosis of dementia. As the patient develops his role and comes to understand that he is accepted, he becomes free to develop new friendships. The group spirit and cohesiveness found among patients is striking.

Therapy. Although the treatment offered to the patient with Alzheimer's disease is not curative, it maximizes remaining skills and allows the individual to adapt as well as possible to his continuing decline. To this end, an important goal for staff members is the reduction of inappropriate behaviors. Some patients pursue a vigorous regimen during the earlier stages of the disease, such as occupational and speech therapy. As it progresses, a variety of additional techniques may be used to manage behavioral and cognitive problems, including reality orientation, movement, art and music therapies, and activity or expressive groups.

The Day Care Center

Day care programs are developed because a sponsoring agency has made a commitment to provide a service that is more intensive and organized than simple custodial care. The center has a variety of goals beyond those of patient care, including:

The collection and dissemination of information. Caring for a group of patients over an extended period of time provides an opportunity to collect a wealth of information and data. Sharing this information with other groups having similar interests stimulates the formation of new day care programs and strengthens the overall concept that dementia can be managed through such programs.

Research. One of the most important aspects of a day program is that it permits the study of the natural history of dementing illness.

If patients are properly diagnosed before entrance to the program, it provides a population for a variety of research protocols and possible therapeutic trials. Families are often very supportive of such research, and while it is not always possible to obtain informed consent from the cognitively impaired patient, every effort should be made to familiarize him with any testing done at the center. A practical outcome of these programs will be the development of a variety of therapeutic programs for the cognitively impaired, and staff members will be involved in the study of how day care programs may modify a patient's decline.

Training. A well organized center provides an excellent training opportunity for a variety of health care workers. Training can involve: 1) visits in which individuals can observe the interaction of patients and staff; 2) internship and field experience for students involving direct experience in managing patients with dementia; and 3) the development of written and visual training materials to educate those in the program and the community.

Day Care as Part of a Continuum

Day care is one of many health care options in the continuum of services for the elderly who suffer from dementia. The elderly population and the number of cognitively impaired individuals is increasing, as are advances in diagnostic and other medical services available to them. One of the forces behind the development of programs that meet their needs is the growing caregiver population.

Family members often resist separation from their ill relatives and, when practical, choose to keep the person with dementia at home. Day care offers them respite but also fills the need for care when an individual is not yet "ready" for long term care placement. The day care program can postpone institutionalization both by reducing the emotional and physical burden on the caregiver and by providing training and intervention for the patient. Through local efforts and the development of politically astute organizations, family members and other caregivers are stimulating further development of this health care option.

In some areas, day care programs are one of the few practical options for a family when skilled nursing or health-related facility placement cannot be obtained or afforded. Families also need services and relief from caretaking when long term care placement is pending, e.g. the patient is on a waiting list for nursing home admission.

Why Separate Dementia Programs? —————————

With increasing concern about how our health care dollars are spent, day programs targeted toward any given disease can be controversial. Concern usually centers on whether programs for dementia should be separate, or whether patients with dementia should be cared for in existing or developing programs for the elderly. The reasons for developing programs specifically for those with dementia include:

Estrangement from peers. Well older individuals and those who are physically handicapped but cognitively intact often feel uncomfortable in the company of those with major cognitive and behavioral impairments, although they are generally tolerant of those whose impairment is mild. The individual who is cognitively impaired may also feel a sense of shame or embarrassment. There is no doubt that individuals with mild dementia can be "mainstreamed" into available adult activities in local communities. However, as behavioral problems increase, centers often find that they are neither medically equipped nor properly staffed to deal with them.

Labor requirements. Some centers have programs that mix those who are cognitively normal with the cognitively impaired, and usually find that division into smaller subgroups is necessary. This makes the program more labor intensive and places a greater strain on staff members and resources.

Environment. In our experience, the optimal physical layout in a day program for patients with dementia, which is supportive of their needs and impairment, may be inappropriate for the frail-elderly and of limited use to those who are well.

Specialized activity programs. Staff members are better able to tailor activity programs to meet the needs of a single patient population. Through trial and error as well as research, specialized activity programs for those with dementia are becoming more refined.

Specialized staff. Staff members who work with this population become increasingly more effective in dealing with the cognitive and behavioral problems associated with dementia, and improve their communications skills and level of understanding of the patient population. Such specialized staff members are often more effective in assisting the individual to go beyond the limits of their disability.

The Organization of the Day Care Program —————

Day programs can be developed by a variety of organizations and groups of individuals, each having unique goals and objectives, and the range of sophistication of these centers will be enormous. No one formula for staffing, physical space design, or program planning can be universally applied. However, if an organization plans to develop a day program specific for those with dementing illnesses, it must be willing to embrace new ideas and options rather than attempting to strictly superimpose traditional day care policies and procedures developed in other settings. Regardless of whether the sponsoring agency is a large hospital corporation or a local community group, the possibility of developing new avenues of care for those with cognitive impairments should be explored. Additionally, education must be provided to governmental and regulatory agencies regarding the successes and failures of day programs for those with Alzheimer's disease and related disorders. We must provide evidence that day care for dementia is a practical, powerful, and humane option in long term care.

Physical Facilities

This chapter provides a series of practical recommendations for developing, modifying, or converting existing space to support therapeutic programs for patients with Alzheimer's disease and other dementing illnesses. Those readers interested in choosing a physical site or developing a new physical structure should seek expert advice and consultation before selecting an architect or contractor.

Before any building or conversions of space is considered, several steps need to be taken.

Develop a space planning committee. While "design by committee" can be a long and frustrating experience, it is essential that one group assemble and act on all information relevant to physical space planning. It may include: 1) a representative of administration for any program that is part of a hospital or other larger organization; 2) appropriately qualified technical experts, either consultants or in-hospital specialists, who can address issues of planning, engineering, or architecture; and 3) the program director, who can explain the needs of the patients and personnel who will work in the space to the technical experts.

Determine the services to be provided and develop the concept of the physical environment in concert with your goals and objectives, so that it will best serve the patients, families, and the institution in which it is located. The mission of the program should be clear long before any space is converted. Goals such as having a family support group, extensive training and in-service programs, or research programs will have an impact on both the amount and type of space required.

Obtain the services of a consultant if no one on the institutional staff has the needed expertise. A consultant brings a wide range of experience, and most importantly, a sophisticated knowledge base, which can eliminate many potential problems in planning and designing space. Consultants range from the direct service professional to the major corporate consulting firm. To provide for the best program space, try to find a consultant that blends well with your in-house experience. You should look not only for the ability to provide immediate answers, but also for skill in finding information; you should not reinvent the wheel.

Visit other day programs. Seeing an existing program will be extremely valuable in helping to develop your own plans. If possible, ask both administrative and staff-level personnel what they like best and least about their current physical plant, and observe the patients to see whether the existing layout and design supports the work of staff members. In our experience, most directors of day programs are willing to share their experiences and knowledge, on both a formal and informal basis. If an agency plans to make use of extensive periods of the director's time, some form of compensation to the director or program should be provided.

Monitor your budget and be prepared to make changes in your plans to prevent going over budget.

Provide for flexibility and expansion possibilities. How the space is designed is as important as its size. Each program should build on the successes and failures of existing ones, hence the usefulness of comments from staff members in existing programs concerning useful design features, or features currently missing. Additionally, some facet of long range planning must be woven into the space and design plans. Very few programs specifically targeted toward patients with dementia have been in operation for five years or more, but as more programs gain long-term experience, stronger and more sophisticated data will become available for planning space to meet both present and future needs.

If you will be accepting wheelchair-bound patients into the program, the initial design must insure that all program areas are accessible to the handicapped. Planning guides and written codes are available to assist in meeting their needs. While most patients with Alzheimer's disease and related disorders are ambulatory, planning ahead can save reconstruction or conversion costs at a later date.

Plan to meet and exceed all licensing standards, rules, laws and regulations, both internal and external, from the beginning stages of development of your program. Do not waste your own time, or the expensive time of others, in developing plans that are unsafe, inadequate, or inappropriate. Find a good contact in whatever regulatory agencies you work with, and be sure you have the correct information concerning such standards in writing. Additionally, make a point of checking regularly to see if there have been changes in these regulations.

Design Philosophy and the Day Program Environment

Patients, caretakers and staff members will first measure your physical facility by the overall impression given when they first enter the program area. The space planning committee should concentrate not only on the details of the space but also on the philosophy behind the environment. **There is no one correct design philosophy.** Some programs emphasize a home-like environment, while others rely on a more traditional medical model. Patients currently receive excellent care in a variety of day program environments; what is crucial is how the staff refines the space and uses it as a tool for the therapy they provide. The remaining part of this chapter provides information that will assist with the process of adjusting the physical space to meet the needs of the patient population.

There are four basic types of design for an Alzheimer's disease day program:

- **The traditional medical model** has one or two multi-purpose "activity rooms" and specialized space set aside for occupational, physical or speech therapies or other medical services. Often there is a separate section for dining. In this type of environment, individual and group activities are usually run concurrently.
- **The school-like environment** (which is not synonymous with child-like) in which a series of rooms open off a master hallway. This type of facility is often found in a converted school building or space within a school. The rooms may be either multi-purpose or specialized for a specific activity. Patients move from one room to another throughout the day for certain activities or therapies.
- **The home-like environment,** frequently found in either converted houses or when treatment space has been specifically adapted to look like a home. The number of rooms and size of the space is variable, but the common theme is an emphasis on creating a "natural" environment for patients and staff. Many experts believe that this is the ideal type of space for patients with dementia.
- **The "church-basement" space,** which may be rented or given free by a local church or synagogue or other community service organization, and which indeed is often left-over or underutilized space located in a basement. It may be the only option for center-city programs, where real estate costs are prohibitive. Many directors have found that this type of environment may not be ideal, but that it can be adapted to meeting the needs of their patients.

Key Elements for Adapting Your Space ⸺

The following suggestions are meant to be guidelines to assist planning committees, program directors, and staff members accommodate to and effectively adapt space for present or future programs.

Break up one large room into smaller areas, with more than one multipurpose activity room if possible. This

- prevents both patients and staff from feeling "penned in";
- prevents patients from wandering about on the periphery of a large room and thus not focusing on the group activities;
- allows staff members to temporarily remove an angry or anxious patient without disturbing other group members; and
- most importantly, allows the staff to set up or clean one area without disturbing ongoing activities.

The ideal solution is to design the space to have three or four connected rooms. The space can also be divided by movable partitions, providing the flexibility to increase or decrease the size of a given space depending upon the number of patients.

If major alterations such as walls or partitions are not possible, large cabinets, sturdy racks with plants, or heavy bookcases may provide a sufficient visual barrier to provide the necessary space separation.

Keep unnecessary human traffic to a minimum, since patients with Alzheimer's disease and other dementing disorders are easily distracted. It is particularly important that program activity areas are not needed as through-ways to other space, as the movement of people through a program area disrupts the concentration of both patients and staff; in addition, patients will often try to follow people who do walk through an area. Human traffic is also disruptive when patients observe a regular passage of people whom they cannot identify; for example, if non-program personnel use a corridor just off the program area, patients often want to investigate whether that person may be a relative or the individual who will provide their ride home.

If you are located off a busy hallway, with glass or windows between the hallway and program area, the addition of curtains may help to reduce the visual impact of traffic. A bright poster or sign may also be used to reduce or prevent unnecessary traffic. Most people will understand that the safety and security of the patients is a high priority.

Disguise exits or have multiple doors before the exit out of the building to help the staff prevent patients from leaving. Wandering by patients is covered in greater detail in Chapter 9.

A storage area is needed where a large variety of items can be locked away. A large walk-in type of closet or small room can be used to store such items as paper goods, meal supplies, equipment for music or art groups, a stereo, VCR, or other electronic equipment, seasonal supplies, etc. The treatment areas should not be cluttered, since patients have a tendency to pick up and hide small items, or to place them in pockets or purses. At the end of the day, items such as a coffee or hot water maker, stereo, or record collection, should be locked away to prevent their disappearance. Any article, large or small, that might injure a patient must also be stored. The storage area should be cleaned and organized on a quarterly or more frequent schedule to prevent it from becoming cluttered and unusable.

Some programs combine their storage areas and coatroom; coats are hung on a portable rack in the morning and moved into the storage area to prevent patients from seeing them.

A large storage area also provides archive space in which art or other work done by patients can be kept. If this material is properly catalogued, it will provide reference material to compare with future projects.

A kitchen area is not a necessity, but is a desirable addition to any day program space. Its most obvious function is to permit the development of cooking programs; it will be most useful during holiday seasons when traditional holiday and ethnic foods can be prepared. However, the kitchen area is not often used to prepare the program's lunches.

If you do not have kitchen space, you will need a refrigerator for storing perishables, a sink so that you do not have to leave the program area for simple cleanups, and at least one storage cabinet. If you plan to do art therapy or work on other projects that will get the patients' hands dirtied, it is very helpful to have more than one sink in the program area.

You may find it necessary to lock the refrigerator and kitchen cabinets to prevent patients from taking food or supplies. If you have a stove, avoid using open flame gas ranges, and try to purchase one with burner controls that allow you to remove the knobs.

A quiet area can be used for any activity that requires the absolute minimum of distractions. It can be used by staff members to provide one-on-one assistance to an agitated patient who needs to be temporarily separated from the group, by staff members when testing or examining a patient, etc. If large enough, this area can also serve as a staff meeting room and as a conference room when visitors are present.

Office space for the director and staff should include a private area where staff members can separate themselves from patients during lunch and other breaks, and where the director will have privacy for interviewing and holding staff and family conferences. Each staff member should have his own desk or surface area for private work, and a stack of small lockers can provide safe places for storage of wallets, purses, etc. If the staff offices are not within hearing distance of the main activity rooms, either an intercom or phone system should be installed so that assistance can be summoned when needed.

Environmental Considerations ⎯⎯⎯⎯⎯⎯⎯⎯

Floors must be easy to clean, and cleaned on a daily basis. Waxed floors that produce a glare should be avoided, since they will confuse or annoy many patients, and may become slippery and dangerous if liquid is spilled. Carpets should be avoided; they are difficult to clean and become unpleasant if someone is incontinent.

Windows in the activity area can either be an asset or serious problem. They allow the illusion of freedom, provide orientation to the time and season, and help prevent both staff members and patients from feeling claustrophobic, but a too busy view or scene can seriously distract or even agitate patients. For example, rain or snowstorms may seriously upset patients, who may feel that they need to return home immediately. Bright sunlight may produce a glare that is both annoying and a safety hazard. Blinds or shades are the obvious solution to these problems, but try to invest in attractive, non-institutional drapes and curtains. If you have a large number of windows, a coordinated window treatment will make the area a pleasant one.

Some combination of natural and artificial **lighting** must be arranged. Most programs use fluorescent lighting panels. In areas without any natural light, the use of specialized light tubes or a combination of fluorescent and incandescent lighting can help to soften the quality of the light. Although they add a homelike touch to the environment, lamps that require extensive use of electrical cords should be avoided. Wall-mounted light fixtures can avoid this problem.

Your choice of **wall covering and/or paint** will play a major role in setting the mood of your environment. Wallpaper and other fabric type coverings can produce a warm, homelike feeling, but most day programs cannot afford the cost of purchasing and installing them. Painting is most probably your best option. Specific colors are often not as important in terms of setting a mood as is the number of colors in any room or area. The haphazard use of clashing colors can create a busy, almost unsettling atmosphere, so attention should be paid to how the color of the walls blends with floors, tables, chairs, and equipment. Planning committees should become familiar with published literature on how color affects mood and energy levels, and observe how color has been used in other programs.

The use of orientation cues throughout the program environment is a debated issue. Some centers have large clocks, calenders, or other orientation devices throughout their program space, a concept that can be carried still further by labelling each room with large signs, orientation blackboards in each room, and using color coded lines on the floor and walls. In terms of patient use and recognition, the devices that we have found most useful includes the following:

- Have easy to read, circular clocks in each room. Many patients have some awareness of time, and a clock can be a reassuring device. This is especially helpful when a patient has the wrong time on his watch, as he can be taken from clock to clock to show that "we" have the correct time. Clocks with unusual hands or a too prominent second hand may be of limited usefulness, and patients tend to be confused by digital clocks, tending not to perceive them as timepieces.
- Use a large, portable chalkboard to post the daily schedule in the activity area. The board should be double-sided. If the orientation schedule is on one side, the other can be used for activities, games, etc. Patients occasionally become quite anxious because they do not know where they are. When this happens, the patient can be brought close to the board and a staff member can calmly review the schedule—if the reorientation does not help, often the diversion will.
- A very large monthly calendar posted on the wall provides useful information for patients. Some seem to derive pleasure from looking at it and figuring out the day of the week and date. The actual date can be highlighted with an arrow or circle.

The decision to hang **artwork** in the program area is a matter of taste. Some centers have framed reproductions and posters in hallways and activity areas, which may help to create an adult atmosphere. Many display original art made by patients, but rooms full of art done by cognitively impaired people may give the impression of a childlike atmosphere. On the other hand, some patients do derive a genuine sense of satisfaction from seeing their work displayed, and the decision to display patient art can best be determined by their reactions.

Furniture

When purchasing furniture for program areas and offices, the three features to consider are safety, versatility, and aesthetic appeal.

A collection of tables is preferable to one or two large ones. Tops should be plain, pattern-free and smooth. A dark surface, such as wood or simulated wood, provides a contrasting color to paper, placemats, and utensils. This contrast is desirable because many individuals with dementia have what is termed a "figure-ground" problem, which creates difficulties in visually distinguishing objects that are similar in color.

Tables must be sturdy and incapable of tipping or collapsing. The shape will be determined by the room size, the number of patients, and the activities in which they are to be used. Rectangular and square tables offer more versatility in arrangement patterns, while round ones are useful for activities that emphasize conversation and socialization, such as lunch.

A variety of chairs will be needed. They will be moved constantly, and must be able to withstand a lot of physical abuse. Chairs should be light and stackable, and have a moderately high back and arm rests. Sturdy chairs with metal legs and vinyl coverings are most useful; those designed for use throughout the program day should not be made of fabric, which is easily wet or soiled.

A few large, homelike chairs are attractive, and also allow patients to relax in comfort when they are anxious or feel a need to be alone. Patients should not be encouraged to take naps in these chairs, which might aggravate sleeping disorders at home.

The decision to have "geri-chairs" depends both on the type of patient in your program and possible regulations in your area. These chairs have high backs, are on wheels, and have a lap tray that snaps in place. Most patients in day programs do not need these chairs, but their limited use may be appropriate:

- if you are running a research or drug trial that requires drawing blood or any type of venipuncture, the task can be accomplished in the privacy of the program area rather than taking the patient to a laboratory; or
- in the later stages of dementia when constant wandering may be a problem, they may be used during meal times to prevent the patient from wandering around the program area with food; this should be considered as a last effort when all else has failed.

Most facilities will not need beds in their activity areas. Patients should not sleep during the day, as they tend to wake up disoriented and sleep problems at night may be increased. Sleeping also prevents the patient from participating in the group process. However, some states may require a certain number of beds per number of patients, which should be determined by checking with the appropriate agency.

Sturdy metal or wooden wheeled carts are a valuable addition.

They are especially useful when staff members must transport items such as a stereo, exercise equipment, instruments, or bulky supplies from room to room.

Safety

Due to the diminished capacity of the patients to perceive their environment, plus possible age-related physical changes or disorders, staff members should pay special attention to the following potential hazards:

- **Glass doors and large windows;** the experience of having someone injure themselves because they "did not see" the glass can be reduced or eliminated by the use of designs or markers on the glass, or by using curtains. All windows should be fitted with locks, and should be repaired if they have a tendency to close quickly or slam shut. If there are windows in the bathroom, the locks must be secured to prevent patients from climbing out the window to leave the program. Simple maintenance and periodic checks can help to prevent a tragedy.
- **Uneven floor surfaces** must be eliminated to minimize the incidence of patient falls, and small steps or dramatic changes in floor surface texture between rooms should be avoided. Cracks, holes or buckles between tiles in the flooring must be immediately repaired, as patients may not perceive them. Scatter or throw rugs are a major hazard and must be avoided.
- **Clutter and inappropriate furniture,** such as items with a protruding base, small step stools, or small trash cans, add to the risk of tripping or falling. Patients will walk and wander in the treatment area, and the removal of clutter on the floor will help prevent injuries.
- **Inflammable supplies** must be kept in a secure and labeled area and not scattered throughout the program area. Safety equipment such as fire extinguishers and fire blankets should be kept in the kitchen and activity areas.
- **Fire drills,** while a necessity and required by regulations in many states, can be frightening to patients because of the alarm bells and sirens involved. Staff members must prevent unnecessary panic, and arrange if possible for the patients and staff to go to a designated area within the building during the drill rather than leave the building. Such details must be worked out with the administration of your facility, and if necessary with a director of safety or security. If the pro-

gram is not located within or attached to a larger health care facility, a fire drill plan must be developed and approved by the proper local authorities.

Additional Issues in Planning Space ⸻

Access to an outside patio or walk area is a welcomed addition to any day program. The ideal area should have enough space so that the patients can walk and explore without needing to have a staff member constantly with them, although they should never be left unattended in this area. The use of outside space should be part of the structured daily program if possible, not just an easy way to pass time (see Chapter 6).

Noise such as intercom systems, bells, buzzers, traffic, and echoes interfere with the patients' ability to concentrate, and must be kept to a minimum. Certain abrupt and jarring noises, such as a chair scraping across a floor, car horns, or doors slamming, can upset a patient and lead to potentially catastrophic reactions. Such noise problems can be decreased or eliminated through appropriate physical design and staff education.

The **temperature** should be kept constant throughout the program area. Drafts from windows or air conditioning ducts can be particularly distressing, and inappropriate changes in room temperature can result in patients asking for their coats, which then can escalate into demands to go home. Some elderly patients may feel cold throughout the year as a result of hypothermia associated with the aging process, and a supply of sweaters or afghans can be helpful.

Entrances and exits to the building should be located near where patients arrive, and should have a covered walkway or ramp to provide a reliable walking surface, even in inclement weather. Ideally, the program should have a separate entrance used only by the patients and staff.

Consider making program space available to community groups such as local chapters of the Alzheimer's Disease and Related Disorders Association, which often need space for general or special meetings. Offering the space during non-program times can be beneficial for your relationships with the community. All such arrangments must be approved by the director or appropriate administrative personnel.

Staffing

As with most organizations, the success of a day care program for patients with dementia is dependent upon the selection, management, and development of its staff. A cohesive treatment team does not develop spontaneously. Staffing requires continuous attention from program directors.

Day care programs clearly do not stop the decline of patients with Alzheimer's disese and related disorders. Staff members may at best see some brief stabilization, but patients will become increasingly impaired and will at some point leave the program. Any system for the recruitment, training, and management of staff members must address both the obvious and latent issues of working with such a population.

This chapter addresses the crucial issues of selecting a director and staff members, the prevention of staff exhaustion, the use of volunteers, and the role of students.

Minimum Staffing Requirements

Not every program needs or can afford a large multidisciplinary team. There are certain minimum requirements in staffing, however, which can be defined in terms of **job functions.** Some job functions cannot be handled by those without professional training. This does not mean that all of your staff members must have such qualifications, but it does mean that you must have the proper balance of professionals and para- or nonprofessionals if you are to adequately meet the needs of patients with moderate to severe dementia.

The following list of mimimum staff function requirements can be used as a guide. How these functions are met, i.e. who you hire to handle what functions, is dependent on whom you can recruit. It is certainly possible to have one person be responsible for multiple functions, for example an administrator who is also responsible for caregiver support programs.

Administration is discussed in the section dealing with the director. A day program cannot be properly administered without leadership by someone who is physically at the center *at least* seventy percent of the time. This individual is the most visible representative of the program, and must function as an advocate for both patients and staff. The professional qualifications for administrating the day care program are highly variable.

Nursing is a necessity. In this author's opinion, this is the one staff position that *must* be filled by someone with full professional qualifications. As discussed in the chapter on medical issues, all programs must have adequate medical support. The nurse is a key person involved in providing this care. Beyond the traditional responsibilities of measuring weights and blood pressures and dispensing routine medications, the nurse often leads program activities, provides patient and family counseling, participates in drug or research trials, and may provide supervision for other staff members. To be successful in the day program a nurse should be comfortable working with a transdisciplinary team.

Caregiver support is provided by an individual who serves as a liaison between program staff and family members. This person also organizes, provides, or refers caregivers for appropriate individual and group therapy. Due to the nature of this activity and since it may at least in part take place outside the day program hours, it may successfully be handled by a part-time individual or someone with a flexible working schedule.

Leadership of activity programs is most often provided by the program staff. The number and type of staff members will depend on whether those who provide administration, nursing and caregiver support also run program activities. If possible, don't try to minimize staff here, since the bulk of the work provided in day programs is the actual running of activity and therapy groups. If the goal is to provide a sophisticated level of care, you will need both professional and paraprofessional staff to handle these activities.

Auxiliary functions such as cleaning and maintenance are provided by housekeeping services in large organizations, or by an outside service or hired staff in a smaller one.

Number of Staff Members Required for the Program

Looking beyond budgeting constraints, probably the key element in determining the number of staff needed by a program is the number of patients to be served and their level of disability. New programs and those with strict and limited budgets must be creative in hiring individuals to handle all of the minimum job functions. Planning boards must also take into consideration the amount of vacation and holiday time each staff member will receive, and assume that they will use sick time.

Any program that serves 6-18 patients per day and has a daily program more than four hours long must hire, at a bare minimum, the equivalent of four full time staff members. This assumes that each staff member can lead program activities or support a group in progress. Given a staff of 4-7, each of whom receives 2-4 weeks vacation, one staff member will be absent for half the calendar year. Volunteers will be essential when staff members are on vacation or ill.

No specific staff to patient ratio applies to all centers. However, to ensure a safe and therapeutic program and to prevent staff exhaustion and turnover, two staff members must be in the room with the patients at all times. Anything less is unwise and unsafe.

The Director

The first priority in staffing a new day care program must be the director. While titles may vary (director, coordinator, supervisor), this is the individual responsible for the organization, administration, and supervision of the program. At a minimum, the director is responsible for the following activities.

- **Supervision of the day care staff,** providing direct, ongoing management of a multidisciplinary team that includes program and liaison staff, volunteers, and possibly students and interns. Such supervision may be both administrative and clinical.
- **Coordination of daily programs,** through the development and management of structured activity programs that are responsive to the needs of patients and which optimally utilize staffing and physical space.
- **Making personnel decisions.** The director is the key person in hiring, firing, and providing regular performance appraisals of the staff. The director is also responsible for adherence to outlined policies and procedures (e.g., sick time, vacation, rules of conduct) if the center is part of a larger institution.
- **Preparation and delivery of public relations materials, in-service training and consultations.** The director is often the person who communicates the objectives, goals and outcomes of the program to the lay and professional community. He should be comfortable with speaking to groups and have the ability to write clearly and succinctly.
- **Responsibility for documentation** varies greatly, depending on

the institution and state or federal regulations applicable to day care programs. The director may be held accountable for meeting specific guidelines and for preparing documentation.

- **Budget preparation and financial management** may involve the preparation and monitoring of a yearly budget. The director will need to be familiar with the financial aspects of the program that relate to charges, reimbursements, and costs. He may also be required to interpret program guidelines to outside sources of payment, such as grants, foundations, or donees, and to third party payers.
- **Short term and long range planning.** A key responsibility of administration is the development of weekly and monthly goals, as well as to coordinate future projects. Directors have a considerable impact on shaping the outcome of a program.

In addition to these administrative responsibilities, many directors are also responsible for direct patient care. Patient contact and/or interactions with family and caregivers require a number of skills, which include the following.

- **Program and group process** skills are needed to provide supervision and planning for activity therapy programs. The director may lead groups on a regular basis or during staffing shortages, and should have training in therapy or rehabilitation and experience in leading group activities.
- **Patient screening and admission.** Families are often in crisis when they come to a day care center. Directors often have first contact with patients or caregivers and should have the technical knowledge and sensitivity to be able to work with families under stress.
- **Emergency management.** The director may need to coordinate and assist in direct care during medical or psychiatric emergencies, since the typical center staff is small.

If the administrator cannot provide these clinical services, they should be assigned to another member of the treatment team, whose authority should be formalized through job description and title.

No one specific discipline or sequence of academic training is required to be the director of a day care program. It involves managing a wide variety of interrelationships—between program and research staff, patients, families, and members of the community. The director must be able to develop a departmental philosophy and program objectives that will be in harmony with the overall goals of the program. The director effectively sets the "tone" of the program, and it may therefore reflect his personality.

Program Staff

The program staff may include therapists, therapy assistants, activity workers, and aides, all of whom provide direct patient care. Finding, hiring, and keeping staff members who will make a commitment to the program can be difficult. At a minimum, these individuals must be able to:

- plan, lead, and participate in a variety of therapeutic activity programs,
- generate new ideas for the program,
- assist with patient documentation, on either a team or individual basis,
- develop and carry out special projects,
- assist with the patient lunch program,
- participate in toileting activities, and
- assist in supervising volunteers and students.

Screening, interviewing and selecting staff members can be time consuming, and a manager with little or no training in personnel management is frequently responsible. In larger programs associated with institutions, a personnel or human resources department simplifies the process. When such support is unavailable, the director should review published materials on interviewing and take advantage of seminars on this topic.

There are no simple guidelines for hiring staff members, but the following comments should prove helpful:

- **Do not screen solely on the basis of educational background.** Education and training are important, but work and life experience also can be powerful and valuable resources. All aspects of the candidate's experience should be considered during the preselection process.
- **Seek out special and creative skills** by encouraging applicants to discuss not only their traditional strengths, but also what unusual talents or skills they possess. The strength of the program and its activities depends on the depth and variety of the staffs' skills. Multilingual ability, a background in music or the arts, or even unusual

hobbies such as magic, the theater, or other performance-related interests, can be invaluable in developing program activities.

- **Look for past experience in running group programs;** since most of the work involving staff members is accomplished in a group setting, they must have, either through education or experience, a basic understanding of how group process develops. They should be comfortable in leading or coleading groups that may range in size from five to twenty.
- **Select for flexibility.** The ability to adapt to rapidly changing roles and to support other team members during periods of stress are valuable skills, which cannot be discovered easily by direct questioning. It may be helpful to ask the applicant to indicate how they might respond to a variety of situations that have been encountered in the program.
- **Choose staff members that are not limited or bound by a particular profession or discipline.** The individual who has a breadth of experience, and is willing to blend her skills with the strengths of others, will be most useful to the program and patients. During the interview process, watch for the individual who makes a point of what he or she does not do; a therapist who only does the specific therapy in which he was trained, or the activity worker who does not believe that professionals should have to feed or toilet patients, will be of limited usefulness.
- **Screen out applicants who need strong feedback.** Staff members deal with a population that can not provide regular, positive feedback to them. They must understand that their activities will not slow the biological course of dementing illness, and that the work done in the program emphasizes what can be done in the here-and-now.

No amount of screening or interviewing can guarantee that an individual will be a successful team worker. It is useful to have job applicants who are being seriously considered spend time in the program as observers. This is not meant as a test, but allows the applicant to observe both the program and the patients.

Staff Development

A lack of complaints about "burnout" does not mean that the working environment is in good shape. Unfortunately, by the time staff members begin to complain, something is usually seriously wrong. Managing staff morale is an important area of management, and should receive continuous attention. Communication with program workers should not be limited to periods of unusual stress, but should be ongoing.

Staff exhaustion is a major problem in any program for patients with dementia. While not all of the following suggestions are appropriate for preventing boredom and apathy in staff members in every work environment, most of them can be adapted to any program:

- **Rotate program assignments** to reduce boredom. All staff members should be assigned to a variety of activities to provide some variability within each work week; a person who is permanently assigned to run a nonspecialty group such as orientation or exercise will usually begin to complain after six months or so. Rotating assignments is successful only when: 1) sufficient notice of work assignments is given, 2) each staff member fully understands what is required within each assignment, 3) a support system (a co-leader, other staff present) permits the individual to complete the assignment, and 4) a feedback system provides critical comment and aid. Management's objective is to provide a challenging environment that is neither too complex nor too oppressive.
- **Arrange the distribution of work** so that no one staff member is assigned all unpleasant jobs. Program set-up, clean-up, and toileting and feeding the patients should be shared by all staff members. This concept must be made clear during the interview and should not come as a surprise. Program supervisors must identify those who avoid this type of work.
- **Act as a role model.** Participation by the supervisor and/or director encourages the staff to share responsibility for the more mundane or unpleasant tasks. While those in supervisory positions may be uncomfortable with this approach because they feel it blurs or decreases their authority, it actually helps to strengthen bonds among staff members. Do not dwell on the unpleasant aspects of tasks, but rather complete them as efficiently and humanely as possible, so that time and energy are not wasted in assigning each and every support activity.
- **Encourage staff development** through regular in-service training and education programs as well as participation in professional seminars. Program managers should encourage staff members to build on and develop their unique talents by giving them the freedom to explore and develop program ideas and opportunities. Typically, health care workers are not often given the chance to realize their potential, but permitting career growth for the individual will also allow the program to mature and grow. Staff development can be encouraged in a number of ways:

1. Staff members can develop an area of specialization; if possible they should work towards certification, registration, or recognition in their field.

2. Staff members can develop research projects and papers that use some of the program's resources; there is often a large amount of information and data available within a day care program.
3. If possible, provide staff members with free time to develop their area of interest.
4. Encourage them to communicate with other health care workers about the development of their ideas.
5. Meet with each staff member on a regular basis to discuss their progress in program development.

- **Provide for staff retreats** by cancelling the program for a full day once or twice a year. Structured planning sessions permit everyone to examine the program and to question whether there are any subtle or major flaws in its organization and management. Retreats give staff members the opportunity to open lines of communication, to discuss and develop new program ideas, and to critique and analyze the program. Some form of agenda should be used so that all staff members have the opportunity to speak. Non-staff members should not attend these meetings. Retreats may raise more questions than answers, but the process will usually serve as a catalyst.
- **Identify problems** by observing the program when activities are running smoothly. Many managers spend a portion of their time discussing the program with staff members and actively seeking creative solutions to day-to-day problems, but potential problems cannot be identified unless they have a firm understanding of how the system operates.
- **Delegate responsibility.** This goes beyond the concept of delegating *work*. Most staff members respond well to being given some level of authority over a specific program activity or project, and tend to make a greater investment of time and energy.

Volunteers

Professional staff members carry out the technical activities of a program, but the contribution of volunteers is crucial to the therapeutic effort. Volunteers and students should never be considered "free labor" or as an inexpensive substitution for staff members. While most volunteers in a dementia day care program will wish to work directly with patients, some may prefer support activities that do not involve patient contact, such as office work, room preparation, and assistance with research.

The ideal volunteer should have a specific interest in helping those with dementing illnesses, and be willing to make a commitment to stay with the program. To be most effective, the volunteer should be available on a particular day and time; this provides greater security for the patients by being routine and structured.

Some day programs will rely on volunteers to provide the bulk of the work involved in its operation. If so, the following options should be explored.

- Try to recruit volunteers with professional training or expertise. Retired social workers, teachers, or other human service personnel are excellent candidates. Unfortunately, their supply rarely meets the demand.
- Develop intensive and ongoing training programs for those wishing to volunteer in the program.

Relying strictly on volunteers will restrict the number of patients and level of disability you will be able to handle. However, it may be the only option for a center with limited funds. There should never be fewer than two paid staff, to insure that a professional will always be present on each program day. If funds are too limited to hire full time staff, consider the option of a quality part-time program.

While a coordinator or director of volunteers may do the initial screening if your program is in an institutional setting, a separate screening mechanism is needed for the program. The following issues are useful for volunteer orientation; they should be encouraged to ask questions if they do not understand any part of the program.

- Patient activities are designed to address problems of memory as well as communication and socialization skills.
- It is not unusual to be irritated by a patient or something that a patient does. If this happens, staff members will provide advice.
- A new volunteer should listen as much as possible and ask few questions of patients, since individuals with dementing illnesses may become anxious or feel humiliated if unable to answer.
- When helping staff members to run activity programs, a successful management technique is to direct the patient's interest back to the program (group process) if he wanders. Patients often have short attention spans, and need regular reorientation to the task at hand.
- Patients are acutely sensitive to the level of tension in their environment, and a calm, reassuring approach is necessary. It is particularly important that panic be avoided during periods of stress. The volunteer should take his cues from the staff, follow directions, and allow time after program hours to discuss any incidents or problems.
- One of the most difficult times for volunteers can be the patients' lunch hour. Their most important role during lunch is to model ap-

propriate social behavior and to foster communication and conversation, but they may also be asked to assist by serving food and feeding patients. Often they can be of most help, not by feeding patients, but by helping them to start the process, i.e., cutting the food, placing the fork in the patient's hands.

Since volunteers are by definition unpaid, it is crucial that their contribution to the program be acknowledged in other ways. This can be accomplished most simply and effectively by remembering to say "thank you," a simple courtesy often forgotten. A more formal system for volunteer recognition might involve a "volunteer day" or party in their honor.

Some volunteers will be uncomfortable working with this group of patients. As with paid staff members, prospective volunteers should spend a day in the program before making a commitment. Clearly indicate that this is not a test, but a way of exposing them to the program and patients.

We do not recommend having patients' family members or caregivers as volunteers, because a major goal of the program is to provide them with respite time. Additionally, the presence of a patient's caregiver would cause him to remain attached to that person rather than join the other members of the program. It is therefore usually best to encourage family members to do volunteer work elsewhere.

It may occasionally be necessary to ask a volunteer to leave the program. Like staff members, volunteers need immediate feedback when they perform inappropriately. They should be re-evaluated if they create additional work rather than assisting the program staff. You must immediately deal with volunteers with strong personalities that directly challenge or interfere with therapeutic goals, who endanger patients' safety, or who develop unhealthy psychological relationships with them. An open dialog between administration, staff members, and volunteers, will greatly reduce such difficulties.

Students

The presence of students and interns, who come to a program to apply theory in a real-world situation, can be either rewarding or completely frustrating. Students can be effective additions to the program when they receive regular feedback from staff and supervisors, and with a bit of forethought their involvement can be rewarding for all concerned.

Developing a student-intern program requires a specific arrangement with local colleges and universities. Literature should be made available to schools describing the day care program and the role students will be given in it, and representatives should visit the program before the first students. Some schools will require a formal contract between programs and students.

If students are to receive a grade for the experience, this must be discussed at the beginning. Before students arrive, the school should send a description of any formal methods of evaluation it requires, and any formal evaluation that you will use during the internship should be shown to the students and a school representative.

Because of licensure or academic requirements, some schools may require that students be supervised by someone with specific academic qualifications, and many schools have regular visits by a field supervisor. In this case the director of the program must still be aware of the activities of each student in the program, and may act in a semi-supervisory capacity.

The presence of students can be a supervisory opportunity for program staff members, most of whom will enjoy the teaching and mentor relationship. The energy and freshness that students bring to the program is frequently a catalyst for perfecting their skills.

Day care programs that serve only patients with dementing illnesses provide a unique, but specific, type of field experience. The type of patients and environment must be carefully explained to prospective students, since those who want exposure to well-elders or to a wide variety of patient populations may not want to work in an Alzheimer's program. As with prospective staff members and volunteers, students should first spend time in the program to observe its activities and patient status.

Because students spend a limited time in the program, it is important that they phase into and leave it gracefully. They often form strong bonds with both patients and staff, and supervisors should provide some formal recognition to help with closure, in the form of a celebration or certificate of recognition. Students should know that they have made real contributions to the success of the program.

Special Issues in Staffing

Part-time versus full-time staff

The typical day program has a limited budget, in which one of the largest expenses is staffing. Directors must determine whether it can best be served by a full-time staff or by some combination of full- and part-time people. There are both advantages and disadvantages to having part time staff.

The advantages include the ability of the program to have a greater variety of talent and skills, since a larger number of part-time staff members may provide more diversity and expertise. Also, part-time staff typically qualify for few if any benefits, and are often a cost-effective option.

There are also major disadvantages in hiring part-time staff. They may miss meetings and charting sessions, have less of an opportunity to share in-service and other training, and may feel isolated from other staff members. They may not have the opportunity to work with all of the patients in the program, and may miss opportunities to share their observations with peers. A major potential drawback of using too many part-time or per diem workers may be disruption of the program's momentum, so that it consists of a series of treatments or activities rather than a cohesive whole.

Part-time staff members must work on a consistent schedule, since their ability to relate to the patient with cognitive impairment depends on consistency. Directors must make a concerted effort to integrate part-time staff members into the mainstream of the program.

Lines of Management

The team effort can be disrupted if staff members report to a variety of department supervisors; the program staff should report to one management line. The director's responsibilities for planning and program development will be made much more difficult if lines of authority are convoluted.

Informal and Formal Evaluations

A formal evaluation and discussion of performance should be made by supervisors at least once each year. Traditional employee appraisals cover job responsibilities and the employee's strengths and weaknesses. Their goal is to relate job performance to the responsibilities in job descriptions. These evaluations should become part of the permanent record of the employee.

All employees should receive frequent feedback. Directors must be alert to unusual stresses or problems, respond to them, and provide individual evaluations that provide direct information to staff members. No one should be surprised with any negative comments at the end of the year.

Summary _____

The initial success and continued progress of your day care program for patients with dementia will largely depend upon having a dedicated staff. Despite the difficulties, frustrations, and unusual demands involved in working with patients with Alzheimer's disease and related disorders, patients are responsive to an interested and caring staff. Despite the patients' continued decline, staff members can have a positive effect on both patients and caregivers; there is a reward in knowing that you have helped someone, if only briefly.

Admission and Discharge Policies

Admissions to the Program ─────────────

Evaluation

Those individuals admitted to the day care program must be tested to determine that they actually have Alzheimer's disease or one of its related disorders, since a wide variety of other conditions can mimic them. A formal evaluation system is needed to screen out individuals with other medical and/or psychiatric disorders. At a minimum, the following conditions must be met:

- the patient demonstrates some level of cognitive loss or memory impairment;
- the patient has had at least one medical evaluation by a geriatrician or neurologist with a special interest in dementia and related disorders;
- the patient has had recent laboratory evaluations—blood tests, urinalysis, EKG, etc; and
- a psychiatric and/or psychosocial assessment of the patient and family has been made.

Developing a geriatric evaluation service for memory impairment is a valuable community service, and will serve as the basis for referrals to the day program. Not every program will have available an on-site evaluation program. Directors may need to work with local physicians, hospitals, or other medical groups to establish a coordinated service. In return for the physicians' participation and support, patients in the program may be a resource for research.

Since one of the goals of families is to obtain respite, requiring that all potential participants in the program go through standardized testing procedures can be frustrating. The director should explain to families why this information is needed, which includes:

- the testing will rule out other illnesses that might mimic dementia, and identify treatable causes of dementia;
- the evaluation provides *recent* information on both the physical and mental status of the patient;

- the results of the evaluation and tests are the basis on which day program staff can develop treatment goals;
- this baseline information is required for research, if the center is planning to study the natural history of the disease; and
- the evaluation will allow the program staff to better understand how to meet the unique needs of each caregiver.

To protect the integrity of the program, no exceptions should be made. If necessary, short-term intensive family counseling should be provided while the patient is undergoing evaluation. It is far easier to explain to caregivers, outside physicians, and others that no exceptions can be made than to explain why one individual was admitted without testing while another was not.

A representative of the program should explain the center's admission policy to prospective caregivers before requiring that a potential patient incur the cost of any examinations.

Developing Admission Criteria

Admission criteria must be set, and understood by all staff members, before any patients are admitted to the program. The following information will influence the development of the admissions policy:

- the center's goals and objectives;
- the availability of staff and physical space;
- the level of cognitive impairment of the patients;
- the size of the program, i.e. the number of patients attending each day;
- the level of behavior problems in the patients; and
- incontinence.

No two programs will develop the same set of goals and objectives. The key is to be consistent in your admissions criteria and to develop a policy that will not screen out patients who are appropriate for the program.

Admission criteria can be kept simple when a good evaluation program is in place. For example, the admission criteria for the program at the Burke Rehabilitation Center are that the patient must:

- have a diagnosis of dementing illness;
- be evaluated by the Geriatric Evaluation Service;
- have some capacity for socialization; and
- be ambulatory.

These criteria allow maximum flexibility and do not screen out possible good patients for the program.

Family and Patient Interviews

The final stage of the admission process is an interview between the program director, the patient, and the caregiver. It begins the patient's adaptation to the program, and there should be ample time for an unhurried meeting. It will:

- allow the director to make formal contact with both patient and family; patients with mild to moderate dementia may have some carryover to the first day in the program;
- provide an opportunity to explain policy, procedures, charges, etc.; both caregivers and patients may have a variety of questions;
- allow a brief assessment of the patient, including general state of health, level of anxiety, and mood; this is the time to find out if the patient has any unusual dietary or medical requirements, and to obtain information that might ease the transition into the program, such as nicknames, hobbies, or other interests that will assist staff members in making the patient more comfortable;
- let the families know the limitations of the program, and that it does not replace primary care or specialty medical assistance; the caregiver must understand the role of the day program staff should an emergency arise; and
- allow discussion of the feelings associated with leaving a relative at a day program such as how they should handle the first day; directors should be sensitive to feelings of ambivalence or guilt, and if necessary refer the caregiver to appropriate staff members for guidance.

The Visiting Day

We recommend that each new patient have a "visiting day" before being formally admitted to the program. This technique is helpful to the patient and allows directors to persuade him to join the group. The patient should be told that he can visit the day program without any obligation to join it. Many patients with dementia will perceive the first day in the program as a permanent or overnight placement, but with repeated assurances of family and staff, they can attend without the pressure of a long-term commitment. The vast majority of patients continue in the program after this first day.

No mechanism guarantees or predicts with complete accuracy that a given patient will adjust to a group setting. This trial day therefore also allows staff members to test the patient's ability to adapt to the program, since some errors will be made even with the most sophisticated screening and evaluation techniques.

Whenever possible, only one new patient should begin the program on any given day, since a great deal of attention and assistance from staff members will be needed. It is important for a new patient to become "socialized" into the group; having too many new members at one time can be a major problem for patients and staff alike.

Disasters can and will happen. Caregivers should be advised to allow ample time on the first day, since if they become anxious or rush the patient, he may become too upset even to walk into the arrival area. If this happens, you may want to consider trying again on another day. The new patient needs gentle but consistent encouragement to stay, a transition that can be facilitated both by staff members and by other patients.

Some families have great difficulty separating from the patient, and must learn how to deal with this process. Such feelings should not be underestimated, even if they appear contradictory to what the caregiver verbalizes. Family members should leave the building on the visiting day, since the staff needs to evaluate the patient's ability to be separated from his caregiver. If the family is close at hand, it is too simple to allow the patient to leave with them if any difficulties arise. As with any rule, exceptions can be made, but the family should generally be weaned away as soon as possible.

All caregivers should receive a synopsis of the first day, whether or not they accompany the patient to the program. It is useful to end the day with a brief meeting with both caregiver and patient, and to thank the patient for his participation and strongly encourage his return.

Discharge

The decision to discharge a patient from the program is usually made by the caregiver, since a patient will usually continue in the program as long as family members can manage his daily care and other medical and social needs.

The process of discharge will also be influenced by the center's criteria for participation. The *administrator of the program* must establish discharge guidelines and a written discharge policy, since he is responsible for both the safety of the patients and the integrity of the program. The following criteria may be used in determining that discharge is necessary.

The patient becomes non-ambulatory and requires physical assistance for all activities. The decision to accept wheelchair-bound patients is influenced by the available space and the number of staff members, but the most important criterion is the physical labor needed to move, toilet and feed the patient. If a patient's decompensated status requires that staff members physically manipulate his body for *each* activity, his capacity to gain from the program and its environment will be drastically reduced. Most centers will not have the staffing needed to provide this type of care.

The patient shows assaultive and menacing behavior that cannot be diminished by psychological or pharmacological intervention. Any program for patients with dementing illnesses can expect episodic outbursts of anger and rare occurrences of violent behavior, although the ability to detect and divert this type of behavior before it is marked will increase as staff members become more skilled. Some patients will not respond to staff intervention or anti-anxiety or antipsychotic medications. These individuals must be discharged to alternative care institutions to protect other patients and staff members.

The patient requires full-time attention and assistance from a staff member throughout the program day. Most day programs can provide occasional one-on-one aid, but discharge must be considered when a patient requires full time special assistance from one or more staff members *every* program day.

Staff members are continually unable to contain the patient within the day care facility. This problem differs from the occasional wandering encountered in many patients with dementia, in that these individuals (often nicknamed "runners") regularly attempt to leave the building. Their attempts may include evading security systems, leaving through fire exits, and even leaving through windows. While all patients will have episodes of going-home anxiety, a patient should be discharged if all methods of assistance, diversion and medication do not diminish his determination to escape from the program.

The number of days the patient is absent far exceed those when he attends. The staff should investigate all chronic absentee problems that may be the result of ill health of either the patient or caregiver. If the day care program is being used as an *occasional* "baby-sitting service," the family should be notified that the patient will be discharged unless attendance increases. Our experience indicates that patients never adapt to the program if their attendance is irregular. Each program day is like a "first day," with its inherent anxiety and stress.

Discharge from the program may also be the appropriate response to specific needs of the patient. For example, patients in the early stages of Alzheimer's disease may not be able to tolerate the level of impairment of some of the other group members. Every effort should be made to encourage higher level patients to integrate into the program, including giving them pseudo-volunteer roles. If after a reasonable time period a patient continues to feel offended or depressed, discharge may be appropriate. Attempts should be made to reintroduce such patients into the program every few months or so, as they may become more willing to participate as their disease progresses.

Some patients vary tremendously in their behavior at home and at the center. Occasionally, a patient who is calm and cooperative at home will be extremely anxious, angry, or simply miserably unhappy in the group, a response that goes beyond the anxiety typical of patients with dementia. The day program may be inappropriate for such patients. Unless its main purpose is to provide respite for the caregiver, the program may create stress rather than provide service in such situations.

Many facilities will consider the possibility of discharge when a patient severely disrupts a program. The time a patient needs to adapt to the program is highly variable. Whenever possible, the director should not set up arbitrary time periods for adaptation. Some patients are quite comfortable and at ease from their first day, while others require months to adapt. More realistically, the length of time that you can allow a disruptive patient to remain in the program depends on the number of staff members and the psychological and medical resources available.

Caregiver needs also affect discharge policies. For example, some families or caregivers have ambivalent feelings toward the patient's participation in the program. Some are anxious about separating from the patient, while others feel that only they can provide appropriate care, and appear to sabotage the patient's attendance. Even with family counseling and psychotherapy, many of these families will discontinue participation in the program.

When caregivers have around-the-clock home health care for the patient, the issue for the family is not one of obtaining respite, but whatever social, therapeutic, or psychological benefits the patient can derive from the program. If caregivers have indicated this to the director, the patient should be discharged if the program is only minimally beneficial.

Basic Rules of Discharge

A family should not be surprised by your decision. Caregivers should be informed as soon as a patient begins to have difficulty in the program, as they may be able to provide information that will reduce the extent of the problem. When discharge becomes inevitable, caregivers must be involved with planning the next step. The decision to seek placement in a long-term care facility (nursing home, veteran's hospital, etc.) can *only* be made by them; program staff can only determine that discharge from the day program is necessary. Staff members must be prepared to provide considerable emotional support to family members and caregivers during this process, as well as concrete planning assistance.

Do not make decisions regarding discharge too quickly. Patients can show incredible variability in behavior, and psychological and/or pharmacological assistance can result in dramatic improvement. If the staff can deal with the problems temporarily, the progression of the disease and consequent changes in cognitive status may also change the patient's behavior. It is important not to discharge a patient before all avenues of assistance have been explored, and the mark of a truly successful program is the staff's ability to develop creative solutions to unusual behavior problems. As a program matures, staff members will begin to take pride in their ability to work with "problem patients."

The center's policies should be investigated if an unusual number of patients are being discharged. A major discrepancy between the admission criteria and the actual level of disability in the patient group may be responsible. Alternatively, staff members may be dealing with difficult behavior problems by discharging patients prematurely. Numerous discharges, especially when a program is new, can create a public relations problem. The program director must allow sufficient time to work with caregivers, and should also be prepared to communicate and interpret the center's discharge policies to the community.

Families should not expect the program staff to handle all aspects of nursing home or other long-term care placement. Families, and not staff members, must visit and be interviewed in prospective long-term care situations. They are also responsible for managing prospective home health care aides. The goal of working with families when discharge is considered is to teach them how to take advantage of available services, and to become familiar with long-term health care systems. Many families are confused or unclear about obtaining information regarding health or social services, and some caregivers need regular coaching and encouragement. However, program staff cannot take on the overall responsibility for planning long-term care; this responsibility ultimately lies with the family.

Arrival and Departure

Arrival and departure times can be particularly difficult due to the disorientation of patients with dementing illness. What happens upon arrival often influences the patient's behavior that day, and the ease with which he leaves the program may influence his behavior at home. Like other program activities, arrival and departure times must be structured to minimize patient anxiety.

Arrival

The process of getting the patient to the day care program can be difficult for both patient and caregiver. It may take hours to get the patient up, dressed, and fed, and if it has been a particularly arduous morning he may arrive at the center with a high level of anxiety and confusion. Some patients will be reluctant to be separated from their caregivers, and some caregivers will be anxious about leaving their family member. To deal with these problems, the arrival time must be organized to expedite the patient's adaptation to the program. The following techniques have proved helpful to us in this situation.

Strictly adhere to a designated arrival time, and limit arrivals to a manageable time period. Even with the best of transportation systems, the arrival period may take 45 minutes. Patients should never arrive unless staff members are present to ease the transition.

A specific location should be used as a transitional or arrival area, and families, caregivers, and van drivers should know its exact location. Consistency is the key to success, since many patients have an awareness of their surroundings and will learn through routine that the arrival area is safe.

A designated arrival time serves as a warm-up for the patient by creating a morning environment that is calm, reassuring, and nonthreatening. No major cognitive demands are made, as patients are gently encouraged to leave the role of family member and make the transition to group member. Most will develop a rapport with other group members and the staff.

Assign staff to monitor this "meet and greet" period and promote the process of becoming a group member through reassurance, reorientation, or diversion. The arrival period provides an opportunity to interact on a one-to-one basis, and staff members should concentrate on patients who are experiencing adaptation difficulties. Some may require a tremendous amount of coaxing and encouragement. A particularly difficult patient can be engaged in conversation or temporarily removed from the treatment area, then reintroduced to the group when he is calmer. This managed process of arrival may also reduce patient adjustment reactions during the other morning activities.

Assigning staff members to arrival time provides a valuable opportunity for contact with the patients' families and caregivers and a chance for them to discuss any problems. Staff members can also use this time to assess family status, since intervention with families when a problem first appears can be extremely valuable. This time period often offers a wealth of information about the patients.

Coats must be taken from the patients, labeled, and put out of sight. Part of the transition process involves parting with coats and hats. If they are in view during program hours, patients will want to put them on and go home. All items of outside apparel should be labeled with the patient's name; the simplest system we have found is to attach clothespins with the patients names to their coats. A portable coat rack can be placed near the entrance to the morning meeting area and later moved to an area where there is a minimum of patient traffic.

Background music during the arrival period is helpful, and should be matched to the general mood of the program participants. If patients tend to arrive tired or sleepy, accelerating music can energize them, while more soothing music can be used on days when the group seems anxious.

Non-demanding activities. Cognitive demands of the patients should not be made during the arrival period. It can be a useful time for routine tasks such as taking the patients' weights or blood pressure, but activities that require the attention of the entire group should not be started during this period.

Assessment of group behavior during this period allows the staff to make last minute changes in the program schedule. For example, a highly agitated group may have difficulty with certain activities.

Absenteeism. Families must be contacted when patients do not arrive on a scheduled day, as they may have been dropped off but did not get to the program area. **Families must understand that they may only leave a patient when a member of the program staff is present,** since even a patient with only mild dementia may wander. Vans or other similar transportation systems should be scheduled to arrive during the mid-point of the arrival period.

Departure ——————————————————————

As with arrival, the period when patients are scheduled to leave the program must be carefully organized. After having spent the day in the program, patients are often quite anxious to find their caregivers, and the desire to return home can be particularly strong. Several techniques are useful in reducing the confusion and anxiety associated with going home.

Be consistent in departure time. Having variable departure times is confusing to most patients and disrupts program activities. The time of departure must be reinforced throughout the day, and posted if necessary. All patients should leave at the same time, since they will notice if one individual leaves early and will also want to go home.

Going home anxiety is common in patients with dementing illness. They may express an urge to leave throughout the day, and this desire may increase as the time of departure approaches. This anxiety is contagious, and if allowed to build up will result in a bursting of patients towards the front door at the end of the day. It may be necessary for all staff members to become involved in the last program activity of the day, to help divert this energy into participation.

New patients generally show more anxiety about going home, and anxiety may resurface as a patient becomes more cognitively impaired. If severe going home anxiety cannot be reduced through behavioral techniques, anti-anxiety medication may allow the patient to participate in the group program.

At least one staff member should be assigned to the front door at the end of each program day, since patients can easily wander during the confusion and mass exodus of departure. The staff member assigned to the door must make sure that each individual who leaves has made contact with their family member or caregiver. Some staff members should attend to coats, while others assist patients in boarding their transportation. Even with the best of staff, 15 minutes or so will be needed to complete the departure process. This time period can be particularly hectic when a program is new, but the level of anxiety surrounding the departure period will decrease as the staff becomes more experienced.

Patients should not leave early, and family members should be instructed not to arrive before the scheduled departure time. If someone must leave early, try to schedule their departure between program activities. It is simpler to remove a patient with a minimum of distraction as the group is moving from one activity to another.

Late transportation should be avoided. Families should be strongly encouraged to arrive 5-10 minutes before departure, and to call ahead if they will be late. When difficulties in transportation occur, staff members must provide the patient with constant, regular reassurance that he *will* be going home and that his ride is only delayed. It is best not to involve the patient in a demanding activity, but rather to engage in a one-on-one conversation of special interest to him. If that fails, a diversion such as a snack or a walk is often effective.

If the patients leave by a variety of transportation systems, keep a list or card file with each patient's name, home phone, and the phone number of the person or service providing transportation. Ways of getting patients home when difficulties occur should be worked out ahead of time with families.

Activity Programs

One of the more challenging tasks in developing a day care program for patients with dementia is to design, plan and lead a series of activities that are appropriate, therapeutic and enjoyable. This chapter will be particularly useful to those organizing full-day programs, but the information can also be adapted to those with sessions of less than three hours.

The major goal of the activity program is to develop structured, nonthreatening activities that maximize the remaining assets of each patient. It should have the following objectives:

- promoting reminiscence and memory recall;
- providing opportunities for verbal and nonverbal interaction;
- reducing physical tension and agitation;
- assisting the individual to maintain some autonomy;
- reinforcing self-worth; and
- assisting the patient to adapt to cognitive and/or physical decline.

The activity programs can have a variety of clinical orientations and philosophies. "Busy work" emphasizes activities that stress rote and automatic behaviors but do not require decision making, such as folding paper, chopping food, or cutting coupons. The goal of such activities is to involve the patients in something that makes minimal cognitive demands. Caregivers find that this type of activity is excellent at home. Other approaches stress creative activities. They emphasize being part of a group process and explore whatever "imaginative potential" remains within the individual and the group. Such activities include poetry groups, music, art, and drama. Effective programs utilize both types of activities to accommodate the wide variety of patients' needs.

Activity programs are useful for clinical assessment. All staff members, including those not trained as therapists, will find that these techniques allow them to evaluate patients' physical and cognitive abilities. Monitoring each patient's deficits and remaining skills allows them to plan activities that address the specific needs of the group.

General Guidelines

The following suggested guidelines will provide an overall foundation for the activity program. They do not depend on variables such as the number of patients, size of program space, or type of staff. It will also be useful to consider them before deciding on what type of program to develop.

Structure. Patients respond best when scheduled activities are consistent and follow a routine. Abrupt changes in the program are aggravating for both patients and staff, and should be kept to a minimum. Patients cannot concentrate on an activity if they are confused about seating arrangements, or about who is leading the group. Advance planning permits a smooth flow of activities, and group leaders should have their materials and space organized.

Avoid a childlike atmosphere. The patients are adults with cognitive impairments, not children who are exhibiting difficult behaviors. The environment and activities must be designed for adults; furniture, orientation items, and supplies for activities should not resemble those used in a schoolroom. Patients will immediately sense condescending behavior by staff members, and will be insulted by a juvenile atmosphere. Both verbal and nonverbal communications by staff members must be appropriate for adult patients.

Reorientation. Many patients will require constant reorientation to the task at hand, and almost all will be easily distracted by inner thoughts or external noise. Anyone directing program activities must be prepared to refocus attention when patients become distracted. They have a strong need for such redirection, and can often be reassured, but the necessity for constant reorientation can cause substantial strain for staff members. It is useful to have a coleader or volunteer in the room during activities who is responsible for redirecting the patients' focus back to the group program and process.

Tempo. It is crucial that you work slowly and gently with patients prone to agitation or catastrophic reactions. They may become confused or frightened when information is presented too quickly, and their level of anxiety may increase. The leader of an activity is responsible for setting its initial pace. Adjusting the tempo of a group is a learned skill, and novices will find it easiest to begin slowly and speed up as needed. Occasionally, a staff member may need assistance to calm a group whose pace has become frenetic. A safety net of staff support is particularly important during the first few months of a new program.

Group composition. We have not found it desirable to divide patients into "high" and "low" functioning groups. From an administration perspective, a major disadvantage is the need for more staff and physical space. Clinically, it can be exciting to run program activities for patients with a high level of cognitive function, but it is difficult to run one comprised only of those with the lowest function and verbal ability. As in any group, the patients in a program will have a mixture of intellectual, physical, and emotional skills. The program will reflect this, and reinforce the acceptance of each member. We have been most effective by aiming the therapies and programs to the higher level patients. Commmunication among the patients results in a higher overall level of function than might have been expected. To be most effective, group leaders need to be familiar with the cognitive skills of the patients in the group, and have a sense of their emotional lability.

Reinforcement. Group leaders need to develop skill in acknowledging responses from patients. A classic mistake is the tendency of therapists to reinforce only happy and positive communication from patients with dementia. They may respond to an activity with sadness, frustration, or even anger; to acknowledge the patient as a whole human being involves encouraging a wide range of feelings. Staff members should thank patients for sharing their thoughts and encourage others to respond as well. Patients are aware of and sensitive to the atmosphere created by the staff, and the day program can be a safe place to give vent to feelings in a controlled situation. Many patients are aphasic or have other problems expressing themselves, therefore **both verbal and nonverbal responses should be acknowledged.**

Minimize distractions. Extensive human traffic, blaring intercom systems, and other interruptions seriously disrupt the process in an activity program. The program area must be designed to minimize both obvious and subtle distractions, so that it will be supportive of the activity leader's efforts to focus the patients' energies on the task at hand.

Program Planning and Staff Assignments ⎯⎯⎯⎯⎯

Good activity programs rarely happen by chance. The foundation for any successful activity program is a pre-planned daily schedule with delegated staff assignments, prepared by the director or supervisor. The schedule should support an environment providing continuity of care, not simply a series of treatments.

Daily schedules are most useful when staff members have time to read them and to organize their time and materials. We have found that a weekly schedule, distributed on the preceding Thursday, allows staff members sufficient time to plan and provide feedback. A sample schedule we have found effective appears on page 49. A copy should be given to each staff member and posted in the morning meeting room. This schedule should provide the following information:

- what activities are planned for the week
- the time schedule for each program
- what staff members, if any, will be away during the week

- which staff members will be leading and coordinating each activity
- which volunteers are scheduled for each day
- a list of any newly admitted or soon to be discharged patients
- a schedule of any outside visitors
- general comments or announcements

Assigning staff members. The director is ultimately responsible for the patients, but this responsibility should be delegated to a leader and co-leader during each program activity.

The immediate responsibilities of the **leader** who develops and leads the activity is to interact with patients, foster communication, and act as a catalyst for therapeutic change. The leader is also responsible for setting up the room and for clean-up, and should be responsible for keeping track of the number of patients in the room. Leadership of activities should rotate among the staff during the program day.

In general, the responsibility of the **co-leader** is to support the actions of the leader, especially by re-orienting patients back to the group activity and assisting those with behavior problems. Patients may need to be escorted to the bathroom or become so disruptive that they need to leave the activity. The need for a co-leader increases with the number of patients; when the patient load reaches 15-20, the need for at least two individuals in the room becomes a matter of safety.

At times more than two staff members will be required in the treatment area, especially when a large number of disruptive and physically active patients require one-on-one assistance. Depending on the number of patients who need assistance in eating, three staff members and/or volunteers should be present during lunch. More staff members are usually needed to assist with the increased confusion during a special event or other deviation from routine. It is also useful to have more staff members available during the afternoon, when agitation and anxiety about going home tend to increase.

Many activities can have a rotating leadership. Specialty activities such as art, music, or dance therapy, are often led by specialists in that area, but all staff members can lead a variety of groups throughout the day. A staff member may lead the exercise program, lunch group, and an afternoon activity one day and be responsible for different groups the next. This approach plus rotation of the co-leader role helps to provide sufficient variety without making the work schedule overly confusing.

Ideally, you should have sufficient staff to permit each member some time during the day to be free of responsibility for direct patient care, including time for planning and setting-up specific activities. If possible, no one should lead two consecutive activities. This can be difficult for new and small programs that have a small number of patients and staff members. When a program expands to five or six days a week, with the majority of staff members working full time, each staff member should have several periods each day in addition to their lunch break when they do not have direct patient contact. If staff members are encouraged or required to write for professional publications in their field, it can be energizing to work time for writing into the schedule, and will also allow them to focus their energies on that task. This is far superior to the more common "hit and miss" approach to writing. Supervisors should also be sensitive to time-off needs when staff members are involved in special projects related to the program.

One of the most important issues in scheduling is communicating to staff members the importance of program leadership. Leading a group involves taking responsibility for the safety and welfare of the patients. This can best be communicated if the director models the appropriate behavior by taking turns at leading groups. The actions of a director during staff shortages will go a long way toward demonstrating the importance of the role of leader and co-leader.

Students and volunteers should have the opportunity to lead a variety of groups. Since this requires a working knowledge of the patients' strengths and weaknesses, students should observe how others lead groups. They should always be paired with a member of the staff when leading a group, and never left with patients without appropriate supervision. They may first serve as co-leader, and then progress to leader as they develop their treatment style.

Directors must be cautious in using volunteers as group leaders. Many volunteers have a strong sense of commitment and excellent skills, but they are not permanent members of the staff. If volunteers are to run a majority of the groups, a significant amount of time must be devoted to recruiting, training and supervising them. If possible, volunteers should remain as support staff, while professional and paraprofessional staff lead activities and communicate their experiences in meetings.

Integrating treatment plans into activity programs. An integral part of program planning is the development of activities to meet patient needs. Since it is not possible to provide constant individualized therapy for each patient in a group setting, generalized plans that focus on the overall goals for the group must be developed during staff meetings. Individualized treatment plans are often developed only for those patients with behavioral problems. While this is often necessitated by the scope of the program, staff members should attempt to carry out some specialized treatment plans for each patient; this concept is discussed further in Chapter 13, which deals with charting and documentation.

Contingency planning. When running a six-day program, *all* staff members must have backup activities or projects that can be started on short notice and that will prevent panic or confusion during unusual situations. Such a situation might occur if bad weather cancelled a special planned program, so that several hours needed to be filled; an experienced staff with a full repertoire of program ideas can deal with such a situation calmly and efficiently. If a particular program idea works, a record of it should be kept for future use.

A Plan for the Day

The length of the program day depends on a variety of administrative and clinical issues. Regardless of the length of the program, the beginning and ending times must be consistent. While a longer program day provides greater respite time for caregivers, some families prefer to have their relative attend more days per week even if the hours are shorter. The program should be organized based on expressed community needs. If you are unsure of how long the program day should be, it is best to begin with shorter hours and then expand, since great dissatisfaction and a major community relations problem can result if a program is set up and the hours then reduced.

A balance of cognitive and physical activities are necessary throughout the day. Since individuals with dementia have difficulty maintaining mental concentration for long periods, most programs run groups that last 30-45 minutes. If possible, try to keep time periods for activities consistent.

Regardless of the type of staff in a program, the typical day should include the following activities:

- arrival
- morning meeting (orientation)
- cognitive group
- a physical activity, often an exercise program
- lunch
- toileting
- a physical activity, often involving walking or games
- afternoon groups
- review of the day
- departure

The sample schedule on the next page can be expanded or shortened depending on the length of the program day. Arrival and departure are discussed in Chapter 5; the remainder of this chapter discusses other elements of the day.

Day Care Program Schedule

Monday
9:15   Arrival
9:45   Orientation
10:30 Perception
11:15 Exercise
12:00 Lunch
1:00   Respite
1:15   Walk/Activity
1:45   Music Therapy
2:30   Dance Therapy
3:15   Wrap-Up
3:30   Departure

Tuesday
9:15   Arrival
9:45   Orientation
10:30 Perception
11:15 Exercise
12:00 Lunch
1:00   Respite
1:15   Walk/Activity
1:45   Art Therapy
2:30   Music Therapy
3:15   Wrap-Up
3:30   Departure

Wednesday
9:15   Arrival
9:45   Orientation
10:30 Perception
11:15 Exercise
12:00 Lunch
1:00   Respite
1:15   Walk/Games
1:45   Art Therapy
2:30   Music Therapy
3:15   Wrap-Up
3:30   Departure

New Patients:

Thursday
9:15   Arrival
9:45   Orientation
10:30 Group Discussion
11:15 Exercise
12:00 Lunch
1:00   Respite
1:15   Walk/Games
1:45   Art Therapy
2:30   Dance Therapy
3:15   Wrap-Up
3:30   Departure

Visitors:

Friday
9:15   Arrival
9:45   Orientation
10:30 Perception
11:15 Exercise

Comments:

12:00	Lunch
1:00	Respite
1:15	Walk/Activity
1:45	Art Therapy
2:30	Music Therapy
3:15	Wrap-Up
3:30	Departure

Morning Meeting and Orientation Programs ‒‒‒‒‒‒‒

The morning meeting provides the foundation for the day, and should never be omitted. It should facilitate the development of the group process that began during arrival, and is a warm-up for the cognitive program that follows. Orientation programs vary greatly, depending on the philosophy of the center and the staff. It may take the form of "personal information training," with the goal of retraining the patients to remember name, place and address. A more typical approach is a gentle reality orientation, whose goal is to remind the patients why they are at the center and what is planned for the day.

Techniques. Serving coffee, tea, or juice is a good way to start the morning meeting, since it simulates the way many social activities begin. Both staff and patients are reintroduced to the group, with particular attention given to any new patients or staff members, or to visitors. It is helpful to have a large photograph of each patient, staff member, and volunteer that can be displayed by the leader while corresponding name tags are held up. Orientation programs are inexpensive to develop; the only necessary supplies are a large, *portable* chalkboard on wheels, name tags, and pictures. Some centers display large, easy to read, wall calendars. The orientation format might consist of:

- introducing the leader and co-leader of the orientation group;
- introducing each patient, staff member, volunteer, and visitor, making a point of acknowledging new or "strange" faces, since patients are sensitive to being "looked at" and appreciate reassurance;
- putting name tags on each individual;
- writing the day, month, year, name, and address on the portable board;
- discussing any weather, holidays, or historical events relevant to the date;
- writing the pre-planned schedule for the day on the board and discussing it with the patients;
- discussing current events if time permits;

- allowing time for questions and answers; and
- providing a *short* stretch and bathroom break.

There is no one correct way to lead a morning meeting. Through trial and error, each staff member will develop a unique style. Some will weave humor into their morning program, while others will take a more serious approach. Regardless of the mode of presentation, staff members must present a genuine and warm welcome to the patients. This goes beyond simply identifying individuals to establishing ties among the patients. The meeting can be used for special announcements by staff or patients, such as birthdays or current events. It is the time when the group should be told that a patient has left (through discharge, death, etc.). Many patients will not remember the contents of this discussion, but the staff should try to discuss every transition.

The success of the program depends upon patient willingness to accept and participate in a structured environment, and the morning meeting provides a gentle reminder that staff members are members of the therapeutic community, as well as highlighting both group and individual responsibilities.

An important addition to the orientation board is the daily posting of the number of patients, which serves as a reference point for the staff throughout the program day.

Cognitive Programs ─────────────────────────────

Programs designed to stimulate memory and reminiscence are generally most successful during the morning hours. The orientation program helps to focus the group's energies in a single direction, and cognitive programs take advantage of this level of concentration. Cognitive programs may include a variety of perceptual activities that stimulate the five senses, memories, and the emotional reactions to these memories. Sensory exercises may awaken both new and old ideas, and are time when the patient's cognitive abilities can be measured. These sessions permit two-way communication without fear of rejection or embarrassment for the patients.

Techniques. Developing perceptual activities involves understanding the difficulties and disabilities of patients with dementia. Cognitive groups can address a number of problem areas, including:

- Language and communication;
- The ability to maintain attention and awareness;
- Orientation to person, place, or time;

- Motor coordination;
- Counting and sequencing;
- Object identification;
- Body part identification;
- Social interaction; and
- Perseveration.

Ideally, the cognitive group should be held in the same room as the morning meeting, to reduce distractions and permit a smooth transition. As with any program, patients should be told its name and what is to be accomplished. Staff members must maintain a sophisticated awareness of the patients' reactions to the program, and learn when to challenge the group with intellectually demanding activities and when to use a simpler exercise. Feedback should be elicited from the patients and used to assess the level of activities.

The range of program ideas are limitless. The most successful activities are those that stimulate memories through sight, sound, touch, and smell. Those that emphasize materials relevant to the patients' age, background, and experience will have a better chance of success than those that do not.

Patients must be encouraged to listen to the program leader, and those who tend to wander (either cognitively or physically) must be encouraged to participate. If patients perseverate on a specific topic during a cognitive session, the group leader will need to change the topic or focus of the perseverative pattern in a friendly and nonembarrassing way.

Any instructions by the group leader should be given in a simple, clear, and succinct way. Reading materials should be bold, easy to read, and non-glossy, and people with hearing or visual loss should be placed close to the group leader. Staff members will need to repeat comments and instructions, and the patients should be encouraged to try to remember. The most exotic and expensive of props will not replace genuine enthusiasm and support of staff members.

The reception of a particular program idea will vary considerably, as a function of changing group composition, the number of patients in the group, and their general cognitive level. If a particular idea is not successful, it should be tried again at a later date since these factors may have changed.

Some Program Ideas

This section is not a "cookbook" of what should be done in cognitive/perception groups, since the programs should be an extension of the staff's creativity. The following suggestions demonstrate the range of possible programs that we have found effective.

Group discussions are most successful when the group leader develops a theme, which may involve the home, a particular period in world history, holidays, emotions, the seasons, children, or trivia. Do not hesitate to focus on unusual topics, since they might spark interesting memories if they are relevant to the members of the group. "Weddings" was one of our most successful topics. One of the staff members, who was married in the 1970's, requested that a patient who was married in the 1940's bring in her wedding album, in order to compare and contrast them. Patients tried to find the similarities and differences in the pictures. This program was so successful that it became the theme of the art therapy session later that day. The key to success was the patients' ability to relate to the topic and the strong emotional content that surrounded the pictures.

Poetry groups are also most successful when they have a theme that helps patients focus on a particular topic. The group leader presents a topic and then elicits words, phrases, and sentences from the group. These are then written down in either a free-form verse or are organized by the group leader. The patients are involved in the process and see the final product. The range of topics in a poetry group should not include only happy events; they might also include such topics as death, sadness, or memory problems. Emphasis should be placed on topics that tap the experiences of the group members.

Word games are not used in many programs, because they can be either too difficult or boring. Success in running this type of program is directly related to the energy level and resourcefulness of its leader. Activities such as word origins, opposites, or scrambled words are too confusing for some patients; it is probably more fruitful to concentrate on games in which the majority of the patients will be successful. A good example would be asking patients to name people, places and things associated with a particular city or geographic region. The purpose of the activity is not only to develop a list on the board, but for patients to share the memories associated with their responses. Word games can be useful either as busy-work or as a creative activity, depending upon the group and its needs.

Sound and musical programs evoke a variety of thoughts, memories, and emotions, and can be integrated into a cognitive program in a simple or sophisticated fashion. A tape, either purchased or made of "everyday sounds," is a useful addition to standard equipment. Patients are asked to identify a sound or group of sounds as the tape is played, and to discuss memories associated with them. Playing and identifying tapes of opera, jazz, rhythm and blues, or tapes associated with a particular place or time, such as Dixieland jazz or World War II songs, has been particularly successful. The quality of these programs often depends on a stereo and/or tape player of good quality. All centers should, if at all possible, invest in a good music system. If you do not have sufficient resources to purchase a large variety of records, tapes, or discs, they can be borrowed from the local library or donated by local community service groups.

Special presentations can form the focus of successful cognitive programs. These include recruiting individuals from outside the center, bringing in community resources, or developing a special project that takes advantage of the talents of staff members. We once brought in a representative of a local nature society, accompanied by live animals. As with other group activities, we began by initiating a discussion about animals, using pictures to capture the group's attention. The goal was to build the level of understanding and communication before the animals were presented.

Cognitive/perception programs are a time during which the decline in patients' cognitive capacities can be measured. The leader and co-leader can monitor such difficulties as increased aphasia or apraxia, and the ability to understand sequencing and to identify objects. Staff members must remember that the programs always have two main objectives, to be therapeutic, and to be enjoyable. The freedom to develop new ideas should be encouraged. The center may also develop research opportunities or projects by monitoring and recording the decline in patients, and staff members may develop interesting ideas for papers and for one-on-one therapy opportunities. How far you develop the cognitive program, from leading games to sophisticated behavioral research, will depend on the philosophy of the sponsoring agency or community.

Exercise Programs

A significant body of literature suggests that exercise is beneficial for the elderly. Exercise programs are common in day care programs, and can be led with a minimum amount of supplies and aids. Movement and exercise groups provide a variety of therapeutic benefits for those with dementia, and should be an integral part of your program day.

The exercise program provides a break from the cognitive demands of the orientation and perception sessions. In addition to beneficial effects on muscle tone and mobility, exercise programs release physical tension. Many patients need an outlet for the tremendous amount of energy and agitation stored in their bodies. Providing an opportunity for relieving some of this energy may assist in establishing a more regular activity and rest cycle. Anecdotal reports from caregivers suggest that exercise and movement programs help to tire the patient, thus contributing to a more normal sleep cycle at home.

Traditional exercise programs emphasize physical conditioning, but movement may also stimulate memory recall that cannot be obtained in any other way. Group leaders should listen to patients carefully for verbal responses and attempt to integrate their emotional reactions to movement into the group's activity.

The exercise room. The actual square footage depends on the average daily attendance. Independent of the number of patients, the exercise room will require the following materials:

- Chairs should be light, sturdy and stackable, with a wide base to prevent tipping while the patients exercise. Since most exercises are done in the seated position, an investment in the proper chairs is important.
- A stereo system or other method for playing music is essential, as music is a fundamental tool in establishing and supporting the exercise program.
- Exercise props should include a variety of balls, elastic ropes and dowels to add variety to the program. Patients seem to prefer balls that have some weight, but these should have some "give" to them to prevent injuries from an overzealous patient. Beach balls can be a good addition to your supplies, but they tend to decompress and break. Supplies geared toward children, such as items with cartoons or other youth-oriented decorations, should be avoided if possible. Many companies supply educational and exercise equipment, including more exotic items such as large parachutes, oversized balls, and ropes, which are not necessary but are enjoyable to use.

Most of the exercise program involves an interplay between the leader and patients. Staff members must remember that injuries can occur if the exercises are not properly done, and that what is appropriate in a health club aerobics class could cause pain or injury in a group of elders. Avoid sudden jarring movements, rapid changes in posture, and the forcing of any limb or joint. If no one on the staff has specialized training in movement, a consultation or series of instructions from a local physical medicine, physical therapy, or dance therapy association would be useful. Numerous books, tapes, and slide presentations dealing with exercise and the elderly are also available. All patients must have medical clearance to participate in an exercise program.

Techniques. The room should be set up and organized, with music playing, when the patients enter. If they have sat through two previous cognitive groups, allow time for visits to the bathroom before beginning. Gentle warm-up activities such as tossing a ball, introducing yourself around the room, or breathing exercises, should be used while the group settles in. Rhythmic clapping or stamping are good starting activities if the attention of the group is scattered, since they take advantage of natural and automatic body motions.

The patients should be able to understand the exercise by observing the leader. Exercises that require substantial verbal instructions or cueing may lead to confusion and should be avoided. Leaders should demonstrate the movements while the co-leader or another staff member assists those who have difficulty following.

The novice leader is often concerned about filling the time period. New staff members should be encouraged to develop a personal style. Some prefer a traditional program that emphasizes moving the major muscle groups, starting with the head and neck and working downward. Others may incorporate dance-like movements, yoga techniques or more sophisticated breathing exercises. Patients are sensitive to anxiety, so the leader must be comfortable with the exercises before demonstrating them to the group.

Leading an exercise program with a group of Alzheimer's patients can be frustrating. The patients will vary a great deal in their ability to follow instructions. Sometimes part of the group will not understand the demonstrated exercises, or a patient may finally learn to perform a movement only to continue repeating it while the rest of the group has moved on to other activities. You should emphasize that the exercise program is a team effort, and try to redirect confused patients with a combination of firm coaxing, humor, and group support.

Both withdrawn patients and those who are agitated need special support. The withdrawn patient often complains of being too old or tired, and participates at a minimum level. This behavior may be caused by a variety of problems, including severe disorientation, depression, or inappropriate medications. While staff members cannot focus completely on these patients during every session, they should make one-on-one contact at some time during the session. Withdrawn patients tend to disappear or hide within the group, and the first step in integrating them into the program is to acknowledge their presence and provide direct support.

The excitable or agitated patient is often a significant management problem. At times movement seems to provide a needed release of tension, but at other times these patients misinterpret either your body movements or verbal instructions and exhibit an escalation of anxiety or even aggression. This type of patient seems to be highly sensitive to abrupt movements and loud noises, and is hypersensitive to any form of criticism. **Do not always try to physically deplete this anxiety.** For example, something as simple as throwing a ball back and forth may increase agitation in a patient with dementia to the point where he has a catastrophic reaction. Diversion or a walk outside the room may be more appropriate for these patients.

Every excercise program should conclude with some type of cool-down or calming activity. Staff members may want to thank the group for participating and to announce the next activity.

Lunch Programs

Any day program lasting longer than three hours will serve a meal. If not properly organized, what should be one of the most sociable and pleasing events of the day may turn into disaster. Lunch cannot be viewed as a "time-out" for the patients. As with any other group activity, **lunch is a treatment time,** a structured activity that requires staff supervision. The patients' success in eating and enjoying lunch, socializing, and communicating depends on the program staff. As discussed in more detail later in this section, the lunch period gives the patients the illusion of freedom, yet it must be one of the most tightly organized group activities.

The time allotted to lunch depends on a number of factors. In many programs the lunch period for patients corresponds to that for staff. Staff members should rotate the responsibility of being at lunch with the patients, since it involves a great deal of work and is not a substitute for time off.

The successful lunch program is influenced by a number of administrative and clinical decisions. The following areas should be considered before starting the lunch program.

Food services. Many programs are part of health care facilities with established dietary departments. If a food service is not available, the director must organize an alternative method for delivering meals which does not involve preparation by treatment staff or volunteers. While in-house preparation supervised by a professional is ideal, you may need to either contract out meal service or hire a trained cook. Another alternative is to establish some type of "meals on wheels" service to the center. Local laws regarding the consultation of a registered dietician should be investigated.

Unless the number of patients is very small, it would be disruptive to dine as a group outside your facility. Whether you select an in-house service, on-site cook, or delivered meals system, a reliable and organized program must be developed.

Patient participation. The decision to allow or encourage patients to participate in meal preparation is complex. Patients in a large program could not prepare an entire meal, but might prepare one course such as salad or dessert with staff supervision. Many clinicians feel that this type of activity is a natural extension of daily skills, and therefore useful. However, your ability to provide one-on-one supervision may be limited.

A number of arguments can be made against patient participation in meal preparation. Staff members find that lunch is most successful when food preparation is left to others, and variability in patient attendance can sabotage a carefully developed cooking program. The needs of the group may outweigh any gains achieved from patient participation.

Eating area. The lunch area should have minimal human traffic. It should be set up ahead of time, while patients are in another room or area, involved in a program activity. Seating patients and setting tables can be simplified by having all supplies, including extra cups, napkins and utensils, in the room and checked before the patients arrive. It is particularly helpful to have at least one bathroom near the lunch area, as it is disruptive to take the patient any distance to the toilet.

The ideal lunch mimics a family meal, since all patients have memories of eating with family or in restaurants. Using placemats, appropriate utensils and non-institutional napkins will subtly reinforce the idea that this activity requires proper social behavior. Trays, layers of plastic wrap, and milk cartons reinforce an environment that suggests illness and hospitals. Even patients with severe cognitive impairments usually have enough remaining social and daily living skills to participate in a lunch program.

The ideal lunch is served in courses. This prevents patients from eating an entire meal in a very few minutes, and allows them to concentrate on one food or group of foods at a time. The goal is to keep patients engaged for the full time, and a carefully paced schedule is therefore vital. For a one-hour lunch period, the schedule might resemble:

Time	*Course*
12:00	roll, butter, water
12:15	soup or salad
12:30	main meal
12:45	dessert, followed by coffee or tea if desired

Serving the food requires some combination of staff and volunteers, with one person responsible for the overall coordination and serving. It is essential that only a minimal number of people be standing during lunch, and to avoid a frenetic pace. The individual who serves the lunch can handle problems as they arise. The server must monitor the temperature of foods; hot soup, for example, can be hazardous and must be cooled for some patients. The server should, if possible, monitor the overall level of feeling in the room, to help facilitate a social atmosphere and hopefully to reduce the number of catastrophes.

Seating patients requires a bit of tact. Assigned seating is useful for a number of reasons, including:

- to prevent patients who upset or agitate each other from sitting either next to each other or at the same table;
- to permit a staff member, volunteer or student to be at each table;
- to seat next to a staff member patients who require maximum assistance in eating, or need to be fed; such patients should be seated throughout the lunch room rather than concentrated at one table or in one area;
- to place at each table a few patients whose social and communication skills are relatively intact, to help keep the conversation from disappearing;
- to allow patients subject to specific distractions to concentrate; for example, some patients become anxious if seated directly facing a door or window; and
- to assign a patient having a particularly difficult day to sit next to a staff member

It takes time, patience, and a good sense of humor to design an optimal seating pattern for twenty patients. Remember to be flexible and to allow for quick changes as needed. Seating arrangements will also change as new patients enter the program and others leave.

Staff roles include modeling appropriate social and eating behavior, intervening as necessary through verbal or hands-on means, and providing mild stimulation to foster conversation and communication. At times, the simple act of demonstrating a skill such as buttering a roll will permit a patient to accomplish the task. Since individuals with dementing illness can be extremely sensitive to and embarrassed by their lack of eating skills, a demonstration with your own food is usually the best way to provide assistance. Try to prevent any one person from becoming the focal point of excessive correction. For example, if a patient is frustrated by his inability to cut meat, try to redirect and refocus the conversation of the group as *you* cut it. Less anxiety and embarrassment will occur if the patient is not held up as an example. If an individual is not using the correct eating utensil, try whispering in his ear or switching utensils unobtrusively rather than providing loud verbal instructions or corrections.

At times, prompt and tactful assistance will be required. A staff member must swiftly intervene if a patient is about to eat a non-food item or is in any way endangering himself or others. Many crises can be prevented if each staff member is responsible for his own table.

New volunteers tend to be too assertive at lunch, and need to be educated not to rush in and try to correct behavior. Volunteers may sometimes feel useless at lunch because they did not "do" anything, when in fact they made a major contribution by being present at the table and thus encouraging a normal social environment.

Clinical aspects. Strengths and weaknesses not apparent elsewhere in the program day can be observed during mealtimes. The abilities observed in the patient during lunch are very often those needed to maintain an appropriate position in the community. Training and intervention used in the day program can be explained to families and caregivers, with the goal of providing a structure to reinforce daily living skills.

Difficulties observed during mealtime may be the basis of treatment planning for other activity areas. For example, a patient's inability to distinguish between his fork and knife and to use the fork correctly (apraxia) may parallel his confusion in using a paint brush. Lunchtime can also be used to observe any unusual changes in patients, since a sudden inability to eat correctly or confusion over what they are doing at lunch could indicate a more serious problem. A sudden change in one daily living skill may warn staff to expect changes in other abilities.

Miscellaneous Tips

Condiments. Avoid putting salt, sugar, catsup, etc. on the table. Even though this mimics a family or restaurant setting, patients will use these items in excess or inappropriately, and they will also tend to disappear into purses and shirt pockets.

Hoarding behavior. Some patients want to take food and "save it for later." Staff members must always be on guard to prevent patients from stuffing inappropriate food items into their clothes or purses. While a cookie saved for later will probably do no harm, vanilla pudding in a purse is unpleasant at least! One of the most common behaviors is a desire to save the eating utensils, which can be discouraged by quickly clearing them from the table. Reinforce the idea that the "house rules" will not allow them to take utensils home because it is not sanitary. If that does not work, make up another diversion so that the patient will stop focusing on the utensils.

Fast and slow eaters. Some patients eat entire meals in five minutes. They should be served last, or served two small portions rather than one. Others will be so slow that staff members must encourage them to eat, and occasionally patients will be so confused that they must be given one utensil at a time and encouraged to eat.

Alternative foods can be provided for those who are not used to a large noon-time meal. Cottage cheese and fruit plates are a widely successful alternative; they are useful for those who have difficulty chewing meat, are a good choice for those on special or restricted diets, and can be easily stored in the refrigerator. Patients who are too agitated to eat at mealtime can be given a cold lunch later, when they have calmed down and are hungry.

Background music during lunch will help contribute to its success. It prevents an awkward silence when no one is talking, serves as a focal point for conversation, and can be selected to provide either an energizing or calming effect.

Clean-up should be done after each course to keep clutter to a minimum, and clearing the tables completely before serving coffee is helpful. All trash should be thrown into a nearby garbage can, which should be tall with a large opening in the side to prevent patients from looking in or rummaging through it.

Toileting Time "Respite"

While toileting is needed throughout the day, just after lunch is a good time to encourage to go or escort each patient to the bathroom. Approximately 15-20 minutes should be set aside for this task. Toileting is discussed at length in Chapter 8.

Walking

A safe area where patients can walk outside is a major addition to a day program. Except during inclement weather, a daily walk can be highly beneficial. It provides a good change of pace, since it is slightly less structured than the remainder of the afternoon. Outside chairs or benches will be appreciated. Some individuals need a quiet time after lunch, while others need to walk after sitting for an hour. An enclosed patio or walkway provides a sense of freedom, but some kind of visual barrier is needed to keep the patients from wandering too far. All staff members should be present, and should "count heads" on a regular basis. Some patients will need protection from either direct or reflected light, which should be provided as alternative space in the shade and by using hats.

Afternoon Activity Programs _____

Anxiety and agitation will increase in many patients as the end of the program day approaches. Afternoon activity programs therefore require careful attention and planning. As with the morning schedule, they should blend cognitive and physical activities. The ability to concentrate and focus on a pure cognitive activity seems to be greatly diminished in the afternoon. Some patients become extremely agitated, while others require attention to prevent them from falling asleep.

The creative arts and expressive therapies are the most useful therapies for the afternoon activity program. These include, but are not limited to, art, music, dance, and drama therapy, all of which encourage reminiscence and capitalize on remaining skills. Confused and agitated patients may be able to channel emotions in a socially acceptable setting using these therapies, and staff members can clinically assess them by observation of the art process, body movement, or responses to sound and rhythm. The creative arts therapies can identify potential problem areas such as low self-esteem, denial, and impaired cognition.

Perhaps the major strength of these therapies is that they allow patients with language and communication difficulties to express themselves in nonverbal ways. Additionally, most patients find pleasure in participating. These therapies emphasize individual skills, but at the same time stress support and interaction from other group members.

If financially possible, your staff should include therapists who have specialized training and meet established standards of certification in fields such as art, music, and dance therapy. The involvement and dedication of these professionals often allows an average day care program to become a model treatment center. Many administrators view these therapies as luxuries. However, when a program grows to serve twenty or more patients a day, it will need the resourcefulness, skills, and energetic input provided by the expressive and creative arts therapists.

If you are unable to locate or retain a qualified therapist, or cannot afford more than minimal staffing, you may want to consider hiring a therapist as a consultant to train your staff in some of the rudimentary skills.

Art and music *therapy* differ substantially from the simple art and music groups that are an integral part of adult day care. Someone who has an interest in music or dance may not be qualified to use these modalities as a treatment technique. The inappropriate use of any activity, including the creative arts, can disrupt the main goals of the activity program. Staff members interested in learning more about the creative arts and their use with adults should contact national associations for recommended reading and upcoming seminars.

Our purpose is not to discourage staff members from working with movement, art, or music. However, if the intent is to provide *therapy* to patients with dementing illness, the best and most qualified therapist available should be added to the staff.

Games

The term "games" is frequently seen to represent useless busy work. However, game-type activities have a real place in day programs for dementia. They are particularly useful afternoon activities on days when outside walks cannot be taken due to inclement weather. Traditional board games and bingo-like activities may be too frustrating for the patients, and also boring to staff members. Games that we have found successful with moderate to severely impaired patients have included:

Charades, in which patients are asked to act out simple to moderately complex daily living skills, hobbies, or other well-known activities. It is helpful to make up cards with drawings of the activity or a picture taken from a book or magazine, since patients tend to repeat the activity out loud if it is described to them verbally. You may need to take the patient out of the room to describe the activity.

Body parts games, in which two patients stand up against large mural paper and trace the outline of their bodies, and others are then asked to fill in body parts. Staff members find it useful to *gently* encourage patients at this game, as it can be threatening to stand before the group and feel as if you are "on the spot."

Modified sports; if you have sufficient space, many sports can be modified for cognitively impaired patients. It is important to minimize the amount of equipment. Avoid those activities that require giving patients a racket or club, and focus on games that involve one or two balls or bowling type activities.

Experiment with games! While they should not be a main feature of your program, they can provide a good adjunct to it.

Additional Group Activities _____

Cooking groups can be highly effective. The sights, sounds, and smells of cooking have a tremendous ability to stimulate old memories, particularly when they involve the preparation of traditional, ethnic, or holiday foods. Not all patients can be involved at one time during a cooking group, so the leader and co-leader need to have backup material ready. For example, while some patients are chopping or mixing, staff members can show pictures of the final product, write the recipe on a large piece of paper, and respond to and encourage memories; it is even possible to write a group poem or essay. It is important to involve all members of the group in the activity.

Group therapy, or group discussion is a structured activity that allows patients to express a wide variety of feelings and emotions. Patients with dementia tend to discuss certain common themes, including:

- loss—the loss of a job, friends, the ability to drive, and most strikingly, the loss of "mind and self";
- questions and feelings about what is happening to them, including feelings of being "sick" or "insane"; and
- anger and resentment, frequently directed at other patients, staff members, family, and society.

Group therapy sessions are also a time to reinforce the ideas underlying the day program. As patients' abilities to find an appropriate word or to express themselves decrease, they can be taught to rely on each other for support.

Staff members often find that the process of getting patients to discuss their problems is very slow, and there is little or no retention of previous themes discussed in the group. They must therefore be willing to encourage patients to repeat previously discussed topics.

Day Review _____

The last element of each program day should be a summary of the day's events, which allows the entire group to review what was accomplished. Many programs serve a simple snack or juice. In many ways, the day review is similar to the orientation program, in that staff members discuss each activity, item by item. The review period provides an excellent opportunity for staff members to discuss any unusual events that took place. They can then remove the patients' name tags, and thank them for their participation in the program. Since patients will leave after the review, coats and hats should be organized by staff members not directly participating in the review program. This time period should be kept to twenty minutes or less.

Medical Issues

Virtually all patients with Alzheimer's disease and other dementing illnesses will have a variety of other age-related changes and disorders, and may take multiple medications. For this reason, as well as the need to manage occasional medical emergencies, all day programs must have adequate medical support, regardless of their number of patients, staff size, or therapeutic orientation.

Primary Medical Care

A nurse on the program staff is often responsible for identifying patients who need medical assistance, is the first person to provide assistance in medical emergencies, and often provides care during psychiatric emergencies. While all staff members must be trained to observe warning signs of illness, e.g., fever, weight loss, extrapyramidal signs, it is often the nurse's responsibility to communicate such findings to the family, the program's medical consultant, and the patient's primary care physician.

Few day care centers can meet all of the primary medical needs of its patients. Unless the center has a physician on staff or in an ongoing consultant role, patients must have outside primary care physicians. The type and extent of medical care provided by the center should be explained to caregivers during the initial interview.

An internist or family practice physician with a strong interest and expertise in geriatrics, or a certified geriatrician, is an important resource for family members. Any health care provider who is sensitive and skilled in the care of Alzheimer's patients could receive a flow of patients from the center, and it is important to identify such individuals through caregivers and other sources.

It is critical that "who" is providing "what" medical care is understood by the program staff, caregivers, and patients' primary care physicians. If a day program consultant prescribes medication, its use should be confirmed by both caregivers and any relevant outside medical personnel. The reverse is even more important—day care staff **must** be kept abreast of any prescribed medical treatment or recommendations by outside medical practitioners. The person who provides liaison, usually the nurse or director, receives input from program staff, caregivers, in-house medical consultants, and community physicians. Direct observations must be added to this information, and used to develop an effective medical management approach, not an easy task!

Program Consultants

Every day program should have at least one medical consultant, who will be available on a regular basis and reachable in emergencies. This physician should hold clinical or charting rounds with the staff, may write prescriptions, and most importantly will be an information resource. A neurologist or psychiatrist is a logical choice, but the most important criterion is that the physician be interested in working with Alzheimer's patients.

Managing the later stages of dementia requires knowledge and skills of psychotropic medication, depression, sleep disorders, etc. The consultant must not only have such skills, but must be willing to use them based on information from the day care staff, who regularly make observations that are invaluable in suggesting the correct management approach in specific situations.

Emergency Medical Care

Any patient may suffer a fall, have a seizure, or develop any number of symptoms requiring emergency medical assistance. The program director must establish a formal system of emergency care for patients; the following guidelines will be useful in doing so.

If the program is part of or connected to a medical facility with an established team approach to emergency situations, **establish an in-house code team to respond to emergencies.** Each medical facility has its own guidelines concerning when it is appropriate to "call a code."

If the program is not part of a medical facility, **establish a relationship with the local police or a paramedic emergency service.** All staff members must know how to summon assistance, with guidelines and appropriate telephone numbers posted throughout the program area, especially next to (or attached to) the telephones.

All staff members should receive basic first aid training, and all staff members, students, and volunteers should take cardiopulmonary resuscitation training and know basic first response measures to take if an individual falls or has a seizure. Staff members should have a basic knowledge of reactions to common drugs, and should be taught to observe unusual behaviors that might indicate the development of a potentially serious problem. If interested, some staff members might be trained in the use of a sphygmomanometer and the taking of vital signs.

Develop a fact sheet or card for each patient that includes name, address, name of caregiver, allergies, pertinent medical information, and regularly taken prescription or over-the-counter medications. This information can be particularly helpful to emergency room personnel.

Prescribing Medication in the Day Care Setting ____

The decision that the day care staff will dispense either over-the-counter or prescribed medications should be made before the program admits patients, as should the decision to allow the program consultant to prescribe medication for use during program hours or at home. This decision carries with it certain responsibilities, and cannot be ignored. The assumption that any patient who needs medication during the day can self-medicate ignores reality, and choosing not to allow qualified staff members to dispense medication will result in the nonacceptance or discharge of otherwise appropriate candidates for day care.

Before deciding whether or not to dispense medication you should investigate the laws and regulations applicable in your area. All states have regulations regarding the proper prescribing, storage, and dispensing of medications, and may also have specific guidelines concerning record keeping. This information can usually be obtained through the licensure and certification divisions of state departments of health. A thorough understanding of these regulations is particularly important for day care centers that are independent of a medical facility.

Once the decision is made to dispense, you will need to establish a supply at the center of medications taken by each patient. Patients should not carry medications from home; it is too easy to lose pill boxes or bottles, and disconcerting to patients to have staff members search for them in pockets. Medications that are used regularly should be kept in a pharmacy bottle labeled with the patient's name.

All drug usage should be monitored and recorded; a clear record of all medications given during program hours should be made by the individual responsible for dispensing them. A chart or index card can be used to list all medication that the patient is presently receiving, and caregivers must be asked to provide information concerning medications prescribed from other sources.

Medications for Behavioral Problems _____

The use of medications to reduce or eliminate behavioral problems in patients with Alzheimer's disease and related illnesses is controversial. The latter stages of dementia may require extraordinary patience, a system of behavioral techniques and the judicious use of medication. When behavioral techniques do not reduce agitation, paranoia, and menacing or violent behavior, the right choice of medication in the right dosage may be the last chance to prevent a patient's discharge from the program. Additionally, it is these difficult behaviors that families find so exhausting, and their control may allow the patient to remain at home longer.

No one medication helps every patient. Each is unique in his symptoms, rate of absorption of drugs, and overall response to a given medication, and aberrant behavior may be the result of a variety of factors, some of which are unique to the individual. The person who prescribes medication needs constant feedback from caregivers and program staff so that adjustments in dosage or type of medication can be made.

This in an ongoing process that must be carefully monitored. Families must be educated to understand that mixing medications—even over-the-counter medications—can cause serious difficulties. When in doubt, the caregiver should check with the nurse or physician in charge.

A variety of drugs are used to reduce behavioral problems in patients with Alzheimer's disease and related disorders, including

- antianxiety agents such as Serax, used to manage anxiety, agitation, and related symptoms;
- major tranquilizers such as Mellaril, which help to reduce severe behavioral problems such as explosive and combative behaviors;
- hypnotics such as Dalmane, which help to reduce bedtime restlessness and insomnia; and
- antidepressants such as Elavil.

Overmedicating a patient may not only result in a toxic build-up of a drug, but also in an exacerbation of behavioral problems. Paradoxical reactions (the opposite of the normal response) to certain drugs may encourage increasing the dosage, which may cause the patient to sleep throughout the day, to become extremely agitated, or to become hypotensive, etc. Such problems can be avoided by encouraging staff members to use drugs only as a last resort.

The success or failure of a drug depends on the caregivers' willingness to comply with the medication regime. Some are so exhausted and drained that they demand medication for the patient, while others may be resistant to their use. It is difficult for most families to accept the fact that their relatives are causing serious disturbances in the program, particularly those who still deny that their relatives are ill. Staff members must make sure that the family understands why the medication was prescribed, what effect it will have, and what side-effects may occur. Power struggles between a staff member and caregiver over who "knows best" for the patient must be avoided. If caregivers choose not to give a prescribed medication, discussion should be encouraged and no anger should be expressed by the staff.

What may appear to be a caregiver's attempt to sabotage a medication regime is frequently the result of confusion or misunderstanding. This is particularly common when antidepressants are involved, or any psychotropic or antipsychotic drug is used; when no apparent results are seen within a few days, caregivers may discontinue the medication without informing the day care staff. Some caregivers decide, for whatever reason, to discontinue all medication abruptly. Education and persistent observation by staff members can help to reduce the incidence of such problems.

The refusal to take medication is frustrating; a patient may take medication without difficulty for months, then without warning refuse to do so. Some patients will only accept medication from a spouse or caregiver, and the occasional patient will believe that you are trying to harm him. The following suggestions may prove helpful in handling such problems:

- If possible, the same person should administer medication every day, as an unusual face may frighten the patient. If the person who usually gives medication is absent, pair the substitute with a regular staff member.
- Find out what makes each patient respond best; some will comply with your request when you use humor, while others will require an authority figure. The person who dispenses medication should be comfortable in assuming multiple roles.
- Some patients may be more willing to take medication when you associate it with a specific family member, e.g., "Mary sent this pill in for you."
- Use the power of the group; if more than one individual at a table needs medication, make a social event out of it. Often a resistant patient will follow the rest of the group when his entire table raises their glasses to toast.
- If a patient becomes extremely agitated, it may be preferable to wait and reintroduce the medication later. This is particularly true at lunch, when agitation can be contagious.

- Adding medications to food or disguising them in juice may become necessary. Be aware that you are in dangerous territory if a patient has paranoid-type behavior, and take care to ensure the safety of other patients. If medication is given in food, the patient must be monitored until it is eaten and the container removed.

Special Medical Issues

Sudden or rapid shifts in behavior must be investigated by staff members or medical consultants. The patient may need medical or dental care and be unable to tell you that he is in pain or uncomfortable, or may be confused over the actual source of pain, e.g., a patient points to her ear and the actual problem is a toothache. As the staff becomes increasingly experienced, they will learn what is out of character for each patient, and that behavioral shifts are often an indication of pain.

Patients who are ill with colds, sore throats, or the flu, should not attend the program. They may forget or not understand minimal hygiene practices, so that runny noses, sneezing and hand contact can easily spread infection. Additionally, ill patients tend to be more anxious than usual, and often are not able to participate in the group. While it may be difficult for caregivers to have their ill family member at home, it is better for both the patient and the other group members.

Depression mimics dementia in its behavioral manifestations, and patients with dementia often become depressed and need medical treatment. Staff members should observe patients for such behaviors as crying, talk of death or suicide, sleep disturbances, or lack of enthusiasm. Some patients who are depressed may appear more anxious and irritable than usual and may develop a pattern of explosive outbursts directed against staff members or caregivers. When depression is suspected, referral should be made to either the in-house consultant or an expert in the local community. If the patient does not respond to supportive therapy or antidepressant medications, he may require hospitalization.

Acute care or psychiatric hospitalization may be a critical turning point in the course of the disease. The drastic change in environment and support systems may produce a decompensation such that the patient is unable to return home, and long-term care placement will become necessary. This is not always the case, and caregivers and program staff should attempt to obtain appropriate rehabilitation or community support services following hospitalization.

Regardless of the medical issue, any change in the status of the patient will have a major impact on the caregiver and program staff.

Many patients are aware that their cognitive abilities are declining, and may also be anxious about their overall health. Whenever possible, families and staff should reassure the patient and provide some hope for improvement. Staff members need to provide support and assistance to caregivers and to pay special attention to patients during any medical crisis. Families need to know that the staff is collaborating with them and not excluding them from any aspect of treatment planning. If a patient is behaving badly during the program day, caregivers should not be made to feel guilty. Finally, management needs to reassure staff that the problem will be addressed, and encourage them to continue providing a high level of support. No leadership vacuum can be permitted to exist when any type of acute medical issue occurs.

Toileting and Incontinence

This chapter discusses behavioral techniques and environmental supports to reduce the frequency of incontinence in day care patients; it assumes that any patient with an incontinence problem has received a comprehensive medical and laboratory work-up to rule out a physical abnormality, disease or infection.

The day care program must have a policy concerning its acceptance of patients with a history of incontinence, and whether or not they will be discharged if they become incontinent. It is a reality of Alzheimer's disease that difficulties with self-care in toileting and possible incontinence will occur as it progresses. Regardless of the policy, therefore, any program that admits patients with dementia will have to train its staff in toileting techniques.

Uncontrolled incontinence places substantial strain on staff members, is humiliating to the patient, and may result in the discharge of otherwise appropriate candidates for day care. Staff members must be encouraged and trained to understand that assisting with toileting is appreciated by the patient and family, and that the patient is an adult with cognitive impairments rather than an unpleasant child.

Our experience with patients supports the following concepts:

- A **consistent** toileting regime, adapted to meet the needs of each patient, will reduce the amount of incontinence;
- It is less stressful, and far easier, for staff members to assist with toileting than to clean an individual who has been incontinent;
- The patient with dementia is aware of bladder and bowel function, but may be incontinent during program hours for several reasons, including:
  - □ he is unable to communicate his needs to program staff, or is unsuccessful in his attempts at such communication;
  - □ he is unable to locate the toilet due to disorientation to the environment;
  - □ the dementing illness has produced a disruption in sequencing and toileting skills, resulting in severe confusion over "what to do" once in the bathroom;
  - □ urinary urgency;
  - □ prescription or over-the-counter medications may have modified his normal body habits.

Toileting Strategies ⎯⎯⎯⎯⎯⎯⎯⎯⎯⎯⎯⎯⎯⎯

The essential components of a successful toileting program are: 1) an appropriate physical layout and location for the bathrooms, 2) the delegation to staff members, and their acceptance of, the responsibility for toileting; and 3) the use by staff members of appropriate behavioral techniques for toileting.

Bathrooms should be located adjacent or close to the activity areas, and more than one will be needed. This is particularly important during times of high usage such as after lunch or before going home. The rooms should be large enough for three people, since patients will occasionally require the assistance of two staff members, and they should be sufficiently roomy so that the patient does not feel penned-in and threatened.

Equipment should be simple, neither too ornate nor too "high-tech," and must include a sink and a toilet with hand rails for support. Urinals attached to the wall may be appropriate if there is sufficient space. Since soap and paper towel dispensers can be frustrating to those with dementia, it may be helpful to place one or two towels on the sink. For refuse, a tall trash can with a swing-type closable lid should be provided; small, round trash cans may be used by patients for urination or defecation. A folding chair is useful for changing patients who do not want to sit on the toilet. Some type of lockable cabinet is useful for storing supplies such as hand towels, diapers, and changes of underwear and clothes. As discussed in detail below, staff members often need to monitor patients' behavior in toileting. You might consider installing doors that are split; they can be opened as one piece, but the slit in the middle allows the patient to be observed without major intrusion. There must be no lock on the door, as patients could easily become trapped inside.

Some type of alarm may also be useful in the bathroom, such as a wall switch that activates a buzzer system, placed outside of the ordinary line of sight. This is particularly useful when additional help is needed with a patient.

The responsibility for toileting must be worked out in detail before patients are admitted, since left to chance and volunteerism, toileting will not be done properly and the incidence of incontinence will increase. Many facilities assign toileting to aides or to the nurse on duty. When assigned to one or two individuals, or to the nurse or an aide, toileting eighteen or more patients requires considerable time. It also produces staff frustration and exhaustion.

A more egalitarian system is the most efficient, in which all staff members, professional, paraprofessional, and other, share the responsibilities for toileting patients. To be a member of the team means sharing both the creative activities and the less appealing aspects of running the program. Assisting a cognitively impaired patient to the bathroom and helping as needed is not as traumatic as most would assume. Additionally, in those institutions that treat toileting and occasional incontinence as routine work, many staff members develop a sense of pride in their ability to meet the patients' needs and see themselves as health care professionals who treat the entire spectrum of problems related to dementia.

If you adopt this philosophy, the fastest and most efficient way to train staff is for the supervisor and/or director of the program to model the appropriate behavior and to encourage discussion regarding toileting techniques and incontinence. Toileting patients should be a part of the job descriptions for all staff members and must be explained to new applicants.

A regular toileting schedule must be developed, and should be discreetly posted in the main treatment or lunch area. The purpose of this schedule is to monitor who has been to the toilet and when. A checklist avoids toileting patients who have previously been taken by another staff member. A staff member should be assigned, on a rotating basis, the job of coordinating the list each day. That individual receives information from other staff members and makes sure that each patient has been given the opportunity to use the toilet. New lists can be posted monthly, and old ones should be saved as a permanent record as they may provide useful research data.

Some patients will require toileting before leaving for the day, and a reminder list for afternoon toileting may be necessary. It is important to prevent patients from arriving home wet.

Behavioral Techniques ───────────────────────────

Behavioral techniques are needed for patients with more advanced dementia. Patients have little difficulty with bathroom activities in the initial stages of dementia, but problems begin to arise when social graces are still intact but the ability to sequence necesary behaviors in toileting is impaired. It is not unusual to observe what appears to be an independent individual enter the bathroom, fiddle with the paper towels or water, and leave, announcing that he is finished. The first stage of intervention for any patient is therefore simple observation. Strategies for toileting the patient will change as the dementia progresses. A given patient's ability to toilet himself will vary greatly, and staff members should be prepared for unexpected changes in the patient's needs and behaviors.

The following sequence of strategies is a working framework that illustrates the complex behaviors involved in toileting patients; it is not meant to indicate that a patient will need each at a specific stage.

Verbal prompts are usually the first techniques used by staff members. Verbal cueing and reminders will assist patients who are independent to locate an unoccupied bathroom. Simple statements such as, "Do you need to use the men's room?" or "This bathroom is empty, please go in," are often sufficient. This should be done on a one-on-one basis; shouting "who needs the toilet" can be embarrassing for all. Patients should be monitored on a regular basis even though they appear independent. Special attention should be paid to the time spent in the toilet, as an unusual length of time may indicate some difficulty.

Patients with this level of impairment are very sensitive to the reactions of staff members, and will also notice the disabilities experienced by others. On rare occasions, those with less impairment may mock or criticize those who have become incontinent. Staff members must learn not to respond to this situation with anger, but to attempt to minimize such comments by discussing with the higher functioning patients concepts of compassion for those who are ill.

Verbal cues accompanied by physical prompts will be needed as dementia progresses. Patients may need to be led to the bathroom and given verbal directions. For example, you should lead the patient to the bathroom, point to the toilet, and say, "Here is the toilet." As adults and therapists, we have been trained to use words such as "urinate" or "defecate." However, our experience has shown that the use of slang expressions such as "take a leak" or "it's time to pee" are extremely successful. Staff members must carefully match the use of such words to the appropriate patient, and they should be reserved for the privacy of the bathroom.

Due to their socialization and conditioning, demonstrations of urination can be very effective with male patients. In a larger bathroom, it is not unusual for there to be two or three patients at the same time, especially after lunch. The visual reminders provided by observing another patient urinating may provide sufficient cues to complete the necessary behaviors. Staff members must be present to reinforce these behaviors.

The bathroom checklist must be carefully monitored, since many patients at this level will either refuse to use the toilet or insist that they do not need it. Some will be reluctant to use any toilet except one at home. Staff members will need to use gentle but firm reminders, and may need to escort the patient to the toilet two or three times.

Hands-on assistance will eventually be required; the patient must be led to the toilet and assisted with undressing, sitting, the use of toilet paper, and redressing. These individuals often take up more staff time than those who wear diapers. At this level of function, a patient can easily misunderstand or misinterpret directions. Staff members must move slowly and talk with the patient while in the bathroom. It is not unusual for patients to begin redressing themselves while still urinating; the automatic behaviors of pulling up underwear or zippers may be so strong that staff members cannot stop the process. You may need to begin again, and re-toilet the patient.

These patients may misinterpret hands-on assistance by staff members as physical or sexual assault. If the patient becomes very angry, the diversion of having a new staff member enter the bathroom will often help. However, there will be times when the patient must be taken into the hallway, walked around for a few minutes, and a return visit to the toilet made later.

Patients at this level may have difficulty with buttons, zippers, or unusual fasteners. Long underwear, complex girdles, or any unusual clothes can sabotage the toileting regimen. The simpler it is to undress, the easier it will be to toilet a patient.

Finally, **total assistance** will be needed by some patients. At this point, the patient may be wearing pads or diapers, and staff members must be prepared to change him as often as necessary. If he is still able to sit on the toilet, a toileting schedule should be attempted. It is important to get information from the patient's family about recent bowel movements, or any changes in bowel or bladder habits. Family and staff members should be aware of fecal impaction, which can become serious and even life-threatening. Some caretakers use enemas, but it is important to seek medical advice whenever unusual changes occur.

Cleaning an incontinent patient is not an easy task. When an individual has an "accident" during the program, he is often humiliated and embarrassed, no matter what the level of dementia. This may take the form of crying, increased agitation, anger, or even physical violence. When a patient is incontinent, he should be quickly escorted to the nearest bathroom, and told what will be done. Urine or feces must be removed from the floor in the program area as quickly as possible. A supply of paper towels and a mop should be kept handy for this purpose. Unless housekeeping staff is instantly available, staff members should do the initial cleanup of floors. Puddles of urine are unpleasant, a safety hazard, and a visual reminder of the incident. Repeated incontinence in a patient within the same program day or over a series of days warrants serious investigation, as a medical problem may have developed, staff may be missing cues, or he may simply need more frequent toileting.

A supply of wet towelettes should be stored in the bathroom to make cleaning easier, and small dry towels, powder, and latex gloves should be available. You should not have to spend time locating these essential supplies. Staff members should always be conscious of proper hand-washing techniques, especially after changing an incontinent patient.

Other Topics Related to Toileting

Changes of clothing will occasionally be needed, and a supply of clothes, including underwear and socks, should be available for this purpose. Caretakers should supply a complete change of clothing for any patient with a history of incontinence. It will also be useful to have a variety of underwear, shirts, pants, socks, etc., to be prepared for an emergency.

If possible, soiled clothes should be quickly rinsed, sealed in a plastic bag, and placed in a paper or other type of opaque bag, since no caretaker will appreciate receiving a see-through bag of dirty clothes. If the caretaker comes for the patient at the end of the day, a brief description of the event should be given. A call home should be made if the patient leaves by van or taxi, as it will be more appreciated than a note sent with the driver.

Toileting patients of the opposite sex is a complicated issue. There is no doubt that both patient and staff are more comfortable when toileting is done by someone of the same sex, but this is not always possible. The patients must be toileted, and there should be no discussion concerning who will be responsible for a given patient in front of the group. It is important not to let anxiety, resentment, or anger build up in staff members. The topic should be considered in staff meetings, and educational films, discussion, and even some role-playing can be used to take some of the discomfort out of the experience.

Diapers are the last approach for managing incontinence. Caretakers may place the patient in diapers after only one incident of incontinence. Diapers placed on a patient too early in the course of his disease will be humiliating and very often increases confusion in toileting. Staff members should also be taught not to respond to every episode of incontinence with the desire to place the patient in diapers. Their use should be a joint decision by staff and caretakers, since once in diapers patients frequently never return to a toileting schedule. Occasionally, a caretaker will give a patient a laxative, and the desired bowel movement will be late in arriving; either very frequent toileting or a diaper for one-time use can be used to deal with this problem.

External catheters, condom-style catheters that fit over the penis, are rarely appropriate for the patient who is still ambulatory. They tend to confuse the patient and are usually quickly pulled off.

Diversion techniques can be a useful adjunct to toileting, but may also be a serious distraction. If a patient is concentrating all her energies on the contents of her purse, she may be unable to pay attention to the necessary sequencing of toileting. Staff members may need to temporarily remove combs, keys, or purses.

The standard technique of running water in the sink or pouring some water in the toilet may be useful in getting the patient to begin urinating. Any system that is helpful should be communicated to the rest of the staff.

Wandering

A majority of patients with dementia develop disorientation to time and space, and a common problem is the possibility that patients may become confused and wander away, or misperceive where they are, and express a desire to be elsewhere. Spatial disorientation and the possibility of becoming lost can occur with a demented individual at any point. It can *never* be assumed that it is safe for a patient to be on his own. One of the major concerns in a day care program is to prevent patients from wandering and becoming lost. The wandering seen in patients with dementia is not usually characterized by aimless or random movements. From the patient's perspective, his actions are purposeful. Some of the more common motivations for a patient's desire to leave the group or the program are:

- **physiological needs,** which may include restlessness due to a need to use the toilet, or being hungry, cold, or in pain;
- **movement away from a source of irritation,** when angry, distressed, or frightened by either a real or misinterpreted event;
- **the belief that it is time to return home,** which can be prompted by a variety of external factors or by internal thoughts; or
- **escape** from the confinement of the program area and building.

In addition to these "purposeful" wanderings, situations when a patient becomes separated from the group and lost may include:

- patients brought to the center outside of the designated arrival time may wander away;
- they leave a bathroom or other room and walk away; or
- they become separated from the group, and wander away when it moves from one room to another.

This chapter does not emphasize the motivational reasons underlying wandering, but rather the techniques that can be used to prevent a patient from leaving the building and becoming lost. Most day care programs do not have locked units. A program that has locked doors can become a fire or safety hazard, so that at best the program should have an alarm or security system. Most of the patients will be disoriented to space and time, and at times their need to walk or leave a room is so strong that on attempting to leave they become assaultive if you try to stop them.

The staff must design the environment and develop diversional techniques and program elements that decrease the chance of the patients' leaving the building and increase the chance that they will remain engaged as a group member. Wandering, like other difficulties, may decrease (or increase) over time, and what may appear as an unmanageable problem may disappear within a few months.

Techniques to Reduce Wandering

Counting heads is the simplest and most effective way of monitoring the group. While it may seem unnecessary to post the number of patients who attend each day, especially in a small program, it is a good and effective habit to maintain. Since each activity has a leader, that person should be responsible for making sure that the correct number of patients are present. This is particularly important when there has been a change of rooms, before and after lunch, and, most important, during and after a walk outside.

You cannot lock doors, but you can disguise them. An unlocked door in plain sight is an invitation to leave. Some patients will automatically open a door and walk through it even without a motivation to leave the program. A particularly effective approach to prevent leaving is to place one or more large, colorful dressing screens of the type often found in physicians' offices in the hallway in front of the door. This often provides enough of a perceptual barrier to divert the patient. However, this may be seen as a safety hazard, and should be checked with the appropriate authorities. Painting a mural on a door that extends to nearby walls also helps to prevent the patient from realizing it is a door. Putting up "wet paint" or "stop" signs may also help to divert a patient. In addition to a variety of visual barriers, having a series of doors before the final exit from the program area is useful. If the program area has a direct exit to the outside, it may not allow sufficient time for staff members to divert the patient's attention away from leaving. Whenever possible, there should be more than one door before the final exit from the program area. At every door, a staff member may be able to divert the patient from wanting to leave the program, and reinterest him in the group program. If your space is large enough, the patient can be walked out one door and brought back to the group via another entrance.

During any emergency, watch the group carefully, and expect the unexpected. For example, a patient may silently slip away while staff members are concentrating their energies on an agitated or assaultive patient. Any time there is a change in routine or the structure of the program changes, the risk of patient agitation is increased which may in turn increase the risk of wandering. If sufficient staff is available, during an unusual event you may want to assign a staff member to each patient with a known tendency to wander.

Reorient patients to the group process regularly. When a patient is walking in the periphery of the group, the leader or co-leader should try to re-engage his interest in the program activity. Staff members must regularly reinforce the importance of being a member of the group. Higher level patients may gain some satisfaction in caring for others, and can use their influence to help re-engage a wanderer.

Monitor medications. Some drugs may increase restlessness. For example, one possible side effect of some of the antipsychotics is akathesia, a motor restlessness that may range from a slight agitation to the inability to sit still. A substitution of medications may decrease this behavior. Medical problems may also increase wandering. For example, a patient with urinary urgency may get up to go to the toilet, forget where he was going and go in the wrong direction.

Post a staff member at the exit from the activity room when you have one or more active wanderers. The staff member should sit next to the door, and divert a patient's attention from wanting to leave back to the activity in progress when one begins to move toward the exit. The ability to distract patients and then re-engage them in another activity is a skill that will develop with experience. One way to do this is to know the patients and their interests sufficiently well so that they can be distracted easily. It is also important to determine whether the patient has a basic need, such as hunger, urinary urgency, etc.

Make a special effort to monitor the group during arrival and departure, since it is during periods when patients are actively moving around that they can most easily walk away without being noticed. When a group gets larger, it will be necessary to have more staff members present at these times (see Chapter 5).

Alarms on doors are used by some centers to decrease the possibility of a patient wandering out of the program area. These devices are usually placed on the doors that are either the main exits from the program area or the exits to the outside. An alarm system involves a risk of being inadvertantly set off by staff members or others in the building, and if such an alarm is set off too frequently it will lose its effectiveness as a warning device.

Educate others in your building to report an individual who looks lost or confused, or who is wearing a name tag or is outside without a coat. If your building has a central information desk, a copy of the current patients' pictures should be available, and the staff at this desk should be instructed to call the program whenever they notice individuals in their area who may be patients.

The Agitated Patient

The agitated or anxious patient is often the most difficult one to divert from wandering and re-engage in group activity. At times a patient may be so angry or menacing that it is almost impossible to keep him in the room. If you suspect that a patient may become assaultive, he should be moved into the hall or another room. The techniques that are helpful in working with an agitated patient have as their goals refocusing energies back to the group program and prevention from leaving the day program area or center.

Learn to detect the beginning of agitation, as it is often easier to redirect patients or help them talk about problems when intervention occurs early. Agitation in demented patients involves a spiraling effect, in which their ability to understand what is said to them sharply decreases as their level of anxiety increases. Patients who are given to wandering may give one or more signals before leaving the room, such as announcing, "well, it's time to go." This statement may be made casually, but an astute staff member will realize it is the first element in a chain of events that will lead to a desire to leave the room; verbal reassurance or diversion at this stage may prevent a full-blown catastrophic reaction.

Try to identify precursors to a patient's desire to leave. This approach involves observing behaviors that occur before the patient actually tries to leave, with the goal of finding out if there is a time period, specific event, or person, that causes or increases the desire to leave. There may be clues that will help staff members to prevent the development of agitation. For example, one patient constantly wanted to leave each day at 2 PM, always pleading that he had to return home. The patient had always had two jobs, and quitting time for the first was 2 PM, when he would return home for a main meal. The strategy devised by the staff was to give a note from his wife to the patient before 2 PM, which explained that he was to go home at 3:30. While this note was not a panacea, it helped to decrease his agitation on many occasions.

"Change of face" is an effective technique for re-engaging wandering, agitated patients. When one staff member is having no success in reorienting or diverting a wandering patient, she moves aside and another moves into place; the "change of face" coupled with conversation is often enough to distract the patient and allow a return to the program. This technique appears to be effective for several reasons:

- The patient is perseverating on the idea of leaving, and the first staff member is part of the perseverative process. A new face helps to break this concentration so that he can be redirected.
- Patients develop likes and dislikes for individual staff members. When a patient insists on leaving, a staff member who has a good relationship with the patient can appear and try to distract him.
- The new person is an authority figure; a staff member who suddenly appears wearing a white jacket and who asks how the patient feels may be a sufficient diversion.

Walking and talking with the patient may be effective. A staff member who walks or runs directly behind a wandering patient can create fear and panic. Unless the patient is in immediate danger, it is more appropriate to plan an intersecting course and to then walk with the patient. Attempts to engage him in any type of conversation are usually more effective than making dogmatic statements designed to orient him to reality. As you develop the conversation, try to physically change direction to lead the patient back towards the program area. By carefully monitoring the patient's emotional state, the adept staff member will know when to use humor or a more serious approach. If a patient is wandering outside the building, more than one staff member should be present to redirect him.

Try to avoid physically restraining a patient who is attempting to leave the program. Grabbing a patient or physically blocking the exit can lead to panic and possibly violence. If a matter of safety is involved, such as a patient wanting to walk into a street or dangerous area, the most easily tolerated technique is for two staff members to quickly link one arm with the patient. Whenever possible, all methods of reorientation, diversion and redirection should be attempted before such hands-on techniques are used.

The Lost Patient

Even with the most highly seasoned staff, a patient may wander away and become lost. The center team should develop a concerted plan of action that can be implemented immediately should this occur. The following approach will assist you in finding a lost patient.

The team coordinator, usually the director or a supervisor, should quickly delegate to other staff and record what was delegated to whom.

This person should remain in one area so that she can quickly be contacted. The leader and co-leader of the ongoing activity should continue running the group and try to prevent any unnecessary agitation among the other patients. The following sequence should be followed:

- **Canvass the entire program area,** including bathrooms, closets, staff offices, etc. Remember that most wandering patients are *not* trying to hide from staff, and that they will often follow the path of least resistance.
- **Assign staff members specific territories** when the search is extended outside the building. Each exit point should be covered, and staff members should check periodically with the coordinator for information and possible leads.
- **Assign someone to make photocopies of the patient's picture,** to use when asking people if they have seen the missing individual.
- **Enlist the help of other hospital personnel** who might be able to provide assistance, and alert the security department if one is available.
- **Write a complete description** of the patient, including sex, age, clothing, etc., and photocopy it for distribution.

After an agreed-upon time interval, notify a senior member of the administration that you are contacting both the patient's caregiver and the police. The exact amount of time to wait before calling the police depends upon your physical location; programs located in the center of an urban area may call for assistance earlier than those located in the suburbs. This time interval should be determined after discussion with the administration.

If police do not come to the center, copies of the patient's photograph and description should be taken to them. The police need to know that the patient has Alzheimer's disease, and that significant cognitive and memory impairment prevents him from functioning independently.

If days go by without finding the patient, contact local newspapers and television and request coverage. Finding the lost patient must take precedence over fear of embarrassing or hurting the reputation of the center.

Caregiver Support Programs

Families are much better able to cope with the distress and frustrations involved in caring for patients with Alzheimer's disease and related disorders when they have access to professionally led individual and group therapies and to family groups led by local and nationally affiliated support networks such as those of ADRDA, the Alzheimer's Disease and Related Disorders Association. The day care program must address the devastation felt by families who watch the mental as well as physical decline of someone with dementing illness.

One of the primary purposes of support programs is to address the caregivers' adjustment to the patient's illness. Each person has a unique set of coping abilities, family assistance, and environmental support systems, and day program sponsored services must be able to respond to a variety of caregiver needs. One of the most common is that families face a growing sense of isolation as social activities routinely enjoyed by them and their loved ones become curtailed. This may be caused by inappropriate behaviors by the patient or a lack of free time due to the almost constant need for caregiving.

Family support programs also help staff members to receive information concerning the home environment, since communication disorders and cognitive impairment often interfere with patients' ability to describe their home situations. Support programs provide a basis for developing an essential communication system between patient, caregivers and day care staff. They also provide the opportunity for families to discuss a patients' successes and failures during the program, filling the need of many caregivers for regular information on what is accomplished in the program.

Types of Support Services

Since each caretaker is unique, no one service or group of services will match every need. Caregiver support can be provided through a variety of approaches, including:

- individual counseling and psychotherapy sponsored by the program;
- individual therapy with a professional in the community;

- a family support group sponsored by the program for caregivers of its patients;
- a caregiver support group led by a professional in the community; or
- a self-help support group (with local or national affiliation) in the community.

While the center staff can provide a core group of family services, it should not require caregivers to participate. Sometimes it will be more appropriate to refer a family member to an outside practitioner for assistance.

Individual Therapies

A caregiver's adjustment to a patient's illness can be addressed by individual counseling and psychotherapy from program staff. Such one-on-one treatment is often requested by family members when they are having a particularly difficult time at home. While this type of therapy may touch upon many issues, it is not meant to be extended insight therapy. The decision to place someone in a long-term care facility or other issues in planning are the types of problems for which caregivers often seek individual assistance from the program staff.

The person responsible for individual therapy is usually the program's social worker, or should be a professional with academic as well as supervised clinical training in individual or family therapy. If no one on the staff has such qualifications, referral to an outside service or consultant should be made.

Individual counseling sessions can also focus on management and behavioral techniques that help reduce behavioral problems in patients with dementia. This type of counseling focuses on practical and basic issues such as the management of incontinence, sleeping difficulties, wandering at night, etc. It can be provided by a variety of staff members who have worked with patients for a minimum of several years and who have developed a repertoire of techniques and behavior management strategies that can be shared with family members. Some of the best advice that can be given to families is information obtained from other caregivers. When such advice is provided, staff members should be aware of the following points.

- Try to help caretakers not to become discouraged if a newly taught behavioral technique does not work, since what works for one patient may not be appropriate for another.

- If a certain technique works at the center, inform the families and have them report what success they have with it at home.
- Not every family member will have the stamina or inclination to develop and carry out behavior management techniques. Some caregivers will not be able to master the skills of managing an individual with dementia. Try to avoid projecting a sense of disappointment when a caregiver is unable to implement a given technique or suggestion.
- Closely monitor the caregiver's behavior during counseling sessions. What may at first appear as a request for management advice may camouflage another painful feeling or problem, which needs to be referred if the staff member is not skilled in the area in question.
- Be careful when giving advice which borders on a medical topic, as giving advice without appropriate medical training or backup is not wise and may be grounds for legal action.

Rarely is any one therapist sufficiently skilled to work with every problem presented by caregivers. Individuals providing psychotherapy and counseling for families should be aware of their limits and refer to other therapists as needed. There will be instances when a given caregiver and therapist do not work well together. Private practitioners in psychiatry or psychotherapy may be the most appropriate referral source for some families. Arrangements should then be made to be sure that all parts of the team work in concert.

Group Therapies and Family Support Groups ——————

Support groups are generally of two types, a family support group led by a professional, either at the day center or in the community, or a self-help group located in the community.

Professionally led family support groups are an excellent way to help caregivers. Some day programs offer this type of service monthly or biweekly, with membership frequently limited to caregivers who have or have had relatives in the program. The group process should be managed by a leader, or possibly by two co-leaders. It is helpful if the person in the program who is responsible for individual therapy also assumes a leadership role in this group.

Community self-help groups are one of the major sources of help for many caregivers. Groups such as ADRDA provide a forum for family members to express their thoughts and concerns, and to share with others their experiences as caregivers. These groups often provide information about new methods of care and research in Alzheimer's disease, and can also help organize talks, workshops, and seminars for both the lay and professional community. Whenever possible, the day program should offer space for these meetings. Because they are usually held at night, there is no space conflict with the program.

Developing a Caregiver Support Group

Most programs will develop a family group for patients' relatives. These are not meant to compete with local support groups, but to augment services already offered. If your program is planning such a group, it will need to address the following issues:

Decide who may attend, by determining whether the group will be open to the general public, to only those whose relatives have been evaluated at the center, or limited to those who care for an individual who is presently a patient. If no other support group is available in the community, an open membership should be considered. Groups open to the general public will vary tremendously in size and membership. We recommend limiting the group size, as many families are inhibited in a large group. To be most effective, a therapy group should have some continuity of membership.

If there are no local support groups, developing a local group affiliated with a national self-help group such as ADRDA should be considered, in addition to organizing a smaller group for day center families. Whatever type of group you develop, the promotional material for it must clearly identify who is eligible to attend.

Consider whether to require attendance. It is rare for a center to require family members to be active in its support group. Most clinicians would agree that this can be counterproductive to both the family and the group, as not everyone is comfortable in a group therapy setting. The more important issue is discovering which type of assistance is the best fit for family and patient.

The format of the group should express the needs and wants of the caregivers. The group will usually become focused on one of the following areas:

- mutual support and growth, a psychotherapy orientation;
- managing the patient at home and in the community;
- progress reports of what has been accomplished in the program;
- new findings in research, treatment, and care of people with Alzheimer's disease;
- planning for the future.

Decide whether to make the group open- or closed-ended. Open groups are ongoing, and individuals may join at any time. People are free to use it as a resource as needed, although regular attendance is encouraged. The advantages of this type of group is that families do not have to wait to become active members in the group support program, and that it is always available to them.

The closed group has a specific starting and ending time, with notice given of when it will begin and how many sessions will be offered. Once the group has started, no new caregivers will be allowed to join. After the specified number of sessions, a new group will be formed. Some believe that this type of group is more intensive and provides the catalyst for a more focused group process.

The level of privacy and confidentiality for the caregivers must be agreed upon before the group begins. The group leader should initiate discussion of whether information revealed in the caregiver support group can be shared with other program staff or whether it is to be kept confidential. *All* participants in the group must agree on whether information presented in the group can be discussed or written about outside it.

The location and time of the group meeting should match the needs of the caregivers. Those programs that serve a large number of adult children of patients may need to be held in the evening or on weekends. The time and place of the support group should be consistent so that families can plan their schedules accordingly. It is helpful to send reminder notices of the meetings to the caregivers of all patients in the program; even if some individuals do not attend, an effort should be made to show that they are welcome.

Special Issues in Caregiver Support _____

More is not necessarily better. While it is critical that every family member understand what resources exist in the community, individual caregivers must decide how they will use day program and outside services. Some families are only interested in the respite services of the day program, and have no wish to join either day program or community support groups. Others find that joining multiple groups and participating in a variety of individual therapy provides a means of coping. Caregivers must decide what service or group of services provides them with the most emotional support and practical assistance. Staff members should not apply pressure on them to utilize existing services. Staff members and caregivers must have an open and nonadversarial relationship.

The new caregiver and the experienced one may have very different needs and agendas. Families who have had access to support services and groups become increasingly capable of coping routinely and skillfully with what once were seen as unsurmountable problems. Individuals who are new to caregiving or recent additions to a support group may become frightened or anxious when more experienced caregivers discuss such issues as incontinence, night-time wandering, or the use of medications. In their zeal to help others, the experienced caregiver may be totally unaware that the advice they give to those less experienced may not be appropriate. The professional or leader of the group is responsible for helping new caregivers blend into the support network, letting them communicate their needs and difficulties. Both staff members and other caregivers can best communicate support through empathy and acknowledgement.

Both the individual with Alzheimer's disease and his family experience major changes in their life patterns because of the disease, and the burden of coping with this change is stressful. The definition of "crisis" is variable, but generally a **crisis** occurs when the caregiver's typical style of responding to change is no longer useful in dealing with a new problem, and they begin to respond in an unsystematic or haphazard manner. Listed below is a small sample of what some staff members and caregivers believe to be major crisis points in dealing with Alzheimer's disease. Often, crisis intervention is sought after the initial appearance of one of these crises.

- the patient becomes incontinent;
- the patient is unable to recognize his spouse and wants the "stranger" (the husband or wife) to leave the house;
- the patient wanders from the house and is lost for more than three hours;
- the patient becomes physically menacing or assaultive;
- the caretaker becomes ill and has no support system available to care for the patient;
- the primary caretaker dies, leaving distant relatives responsible for the patient's care;
- the patient starts a fire or leaves the gas on.

Crisis intervention by definition is short term assistance. For many families, the initial phase of treatment is practical help, e.g., arranging for the prescription of medication, locating home health aides, or hospitalizing the patient. Another goal is to teach caregivers new mechanisms and alternatives for responding to situational problems. Denial among family members may be so strong that only when a crisis occurs do they see that a change in their adaptation to their relative's illness is needed.

The process of **adaptation means forming new bonds and attachment to an impaired individual.** Those who provide family support services need to be aware of this process. One of the most difficult and painful tasks for a caregiver is to accept the progressive limitations of the patient and form a *new and different* relationship to a cognitively and emotionally impaired individual. Each caregiver's response to these increasing deficits is different, and some are never able to reconcile themselves to the change. Difficulties arise especially when the caretaker continues to respond to the patient as if no impairment exists.

When an individual with Alzheimer's disease dies, day program staff can continue to provide support services to the caregiver, although for most of the staff, a patient's death ends their direct contact with the family. Death is a major transition for the caregiver, regardless of the course or length of the illness and no matter how much the disease process altered family relationships. Whenever possible, caregivers should be encouraged to continue with the support programs provided by the center. It is important that this invitation be extended, even though the families may not opt for continued participation.

Transportation

Organizing the schedules and logistics of providing transportation of patients to and from the day care program can be a perpetual and persistent problem. Whenever possible, families should be encouraged to provide transportation. Caregivers are the most reliable and consistent means of transportation, and the patient will feel most secure with family or friends. Not all caregivers can provide transportation; some do not drive, while others have responsibilities of work or childcare. Since a day care program can fail due to a lack of transportation, one member of the planning committee should take on the responsibility of investigating possible alternative modes of transportation.

The methods of transportation chosen will depend on the location of the program (center city, suburban, rural), the availability of van or mini-bus service, and the possibility of developing a transportation system run by the program. The major options for transportation will include:

- walking
- transportation provided by a caregiver
- mini-bus sponsored by the center
- mini-bus funded and organized by an outside agency
- special service, by taxi, public transportation service, or volunteers

Walking

Walking to the day program is rare, since most individuals will not live close enough. In addition, poor weather and the exertion required to walk may be disorienting or disruptive to the patient with dementia. Caregivers should usually be encouraged to develop or organize other alternatives.

Transportation by the Family

Transportation by a caregiver is a common means of getting the patient to and from the program. In many ways it is the most desirable, because:

- the patient is apt to feel more comfortable and relaxed during transit since he knows the driver;
- the caregiver is not as pressured into getting the patient ready on time for a bus or mini-van, which can increase the level of anxiety during the morning routine;
- arrival and departure time can be smoother since it is a direct transfer from caregiver to staff;
- the patient may spend less time in transit; and
- the caregiver is often the best person to provide attention and reassurance to calm the patient if he becomes agitated, or if a medical problem arises during transit.

This system is obviously dependent upon the caregiver, and families must receive instructions concerning safety, consistency and reliability. If the caregiver is routinely late, feels overburdened, and complains about driving, alternative transportation should be arranged.

Caregivers may occasionally carpool with other families, so that drivers alternate days for delivery and pickup. This is something that families should arrange among themselves. Some caregivers would feel very much imposed upon by driving another patient, and it is inappropriate for the center to attempt matching drivers. If family members volunteer to share driving, their names can be kept on file. In practice, however, most families feel that dealing with one patient is difficult enough and do not wish to drive others. The following should be kept in mind should caregivers wish to carpool.

- Carpooling assumes that the patients involved are attending the program on the same days. While this can often be arranged, it cannot always be guaranteed.
- The patients in the carpool must be able to get along with each other and to remain calm during transit. If patients who do not like each other are driven together, arrival and departure times as well as the actual ride can be tremendously tedious and upsetting.
- Carpooling also assumes that each driver share a certain responsibility. Most program directors and staff members do not have the time needed to intercede when caregivers experience difficulties in making driving arrangements.

One of the most distressing problems that develops when transportation is provided by caregivers is what to do when a driver does not arrive to pick up a patient at the end of the program day. While some patients will not mind waiting a few minutes, some become very agitated. When transportation is late, the following steps should be taken.

- The person assigned to the front door should remain with the patient, and should not be assigned other responsibilities.
- The director should assign one or more staff members as needed to assist this person in keeping the patient calm.
- Do not assume that the caregiver is on the way until you contact someone who verifies that this is the case. Call the caretaker's home immediately.
- Every patient should have at least one emergency ride number, someone who knows the patient and will come for him.
- Without exception, staff members should never drive a patient home in a personal car; the possible complications and legal difficulties are simply too great.
- If absolutely necessary, the patient may have to return home by taxi. When possible, a caregiver or friend should arrive in the taxi to assist the patient, especially if he rarely uses taxis and may be upset.

Mini-van Systems

Mini-vans, small buses, and ambulettes can be used to transport patients to the program. The two basic options are for the center to buy a van (or vans) and to hire drivers, or to use an already existing van service in the community adapted to meet the needs of those with dementia.

Vans with fewer than ten seats are preferable to larger ones since travel time should be kept as short as possible. The longer patients are in transit the more likely they are to become agitated, anxious, or even incontinent. Other problems that must be solved before any type of van system can be used include the following.

- Someone must put the patient on the van in the morning and meet it in the afternoon. Most outside van services will not escort a patient to and from the van.
- Some patients cannot tolerate any type of group ride, and will not be able to use this system.
- When a van breaks down, you must arrange alternative services for a number of people. Outside vendors usually have replacement buses to use, but you must be prepared for this contingency if you buy your own.

Having your own van(s) gives you more control over transportation. However, with this control comes added responsibility and costs. If you plan to buy one or more vans, you must be prepared for the startup costs, which in addition to the basic purchase cost may include the addition of motorized ramp lifts or other adaptations. Yearly expenses will include the drivers' salaries, maintenance (which can be estimated as a cost/miles times miles/day), major repairs, insurance, and yearly depreciation. Depending on the number of vans, owning your own may add $35,000 to $150,000 to your yearly expense, which will substantially increase your cost per patient day.

By providing transportation, the center extends its responsibility outside of the physical plant of the day care program, and it will be responsible for the safety and welfare of each patient up to the time he enters his home.

However, there *are* specific advantages in owning and running your van service, including:

- program staff are in control of the scheduling, pick-up times, and coordination of the transportation;
- special trips to pick up a late patient can be arranged without the need to go through a third party;
- providing transportation will be seen by many caretakers as a much needed service, and can extend their respite time by as much as an hour and a half; and
- patients will come to recognize the center drivers, who may then be better prepared to handle behavior problems that may develop.

Another alternative is to adapt and use an existing community-based van system. Such transportation is available in some communities as handicapped, "dollar-ride" or agency-based services. These vary in their ability to meet the needs of patients with dementia. The advantages of using such an established service include the following.

- It is far less expensive to the center than using your own vans, because you are not responsible for costs such as maintenance and insurance.
- Families are responsible for arrangements with the outside agency's dispatcher, reducing the need for staff time to coordinate a transportation system.
- If the patient is comfortable using the van, he and his family may be able to use the service for other purposes, such as medical visits or shopping.
- Since many of these services are sponsored by local area agencies on aging or offices for the disabled, the cost to the patient and caregiver is usually less than the center would have to charge.

If you want to use a community van service, someone on the planning committee or the program director will need to negotiate with the sponsoring agency before the day program begins. Most likely, the coordinator of the service will require information concerning the nature and difficulties associated with Alzheimer's disease. Some van services have age restrictions, accepting only those 65 or older, for example, while others may only accept those with "physical limitations." Almost every community van service will require some type of application process for each patient, which may include a signed statement from a community physician stating his specific needs.

Adapting to another agency's transportation has some drawbacks, which may include the following:

- Families and day program staff must understand that the transportation program was not designed to meet the unique needs of the patient with dementia. These services tend to serve a wide variety of elders and handicapped individuals. They cannot be expected to have a thorough knowledge of dementia and its complications.
- Caregivers and staff must adapt to the other agency's schedules. If the van service does not run on certain days or during poor weather conditions, the patients who use the service will not be able to come to the program.
- Program staff have little, if any, control over the quality of the drivers. While many are excellent, they may have no vested interest in taking particular care with your patients.
- The agency sponsoring the van service may, at any time, decide to stop transporting patients with dementia. Alternative arrangements that can be quickly implemented should be considered.

Adapting an Existing Van Program to Your Needs

Develop a professional and friendly relationship with the transportation coordinator or dispatcher. This individual hears constant complaints about late rides and "no shows." Try to prevent an adversarial relationship from forming.

Offer possible solutions if you have complaints. Most programs that provide shared-ride services welcome positive ideas that help develop better services. The program staff must be willing to take the first step in solving problems.

Develop a relationship with the drivers. Center staff must be willing to provide some brief education to the drivers, and should be available to help patients into the van. Explain to new drivers that these individuals have memory problems, and that they can only be dropped off at a designated site. Let supervisors know when a particular driver is doing a good job, as their merit increases and promotions may be based on this type of feedback.

Be prepared to occasionally bend the rules. If a driver arrives early, you may need to send a patient home before the official departure time. This is disruptive to the program and the patient, but may be necessary, for example, when a driver is sick and another covers for him.

Monitor your patients and make alternative arrangements when necessary. Patients should *never* be put on vans with full bladders or soiled diapers. Patients who develop an acute illness, or are unusually agitated or angry, may not be able to tolerate the ride home. The safety of the patients and other riders must be protected. Some patients may develop an aversion to the van and refuse to enter it. Even though the service is convenient for the program and caregivers, the director must consider whether it is both safe *and* appropriate for a given patient, and make alternative arrangements if not.

If there is to be a transfer of money between patient and driver, be prepared to help with the transaction. Many shared-ride services, for example, charge a minimum flat rate such as $1 per ride. Patients with dementia may become concerned, confused, or even somewhat paranoid about giving money to the driver, while others may be inappropriate in their desire to "tip" him. If the patient has difficulty in money exchanges, have the families send the money to the program so that a staff member can give the driver the correct amount.

Remember that the drivers are not messengers for the center. Do not assume that you can give notes, empty medicine bottles, and bags of soiled clothes to them. Most drivers are willing to help when they can, but they should not be overburdened with responsibilities that are not part of their job. On the other hand, if you have developed a good relationship with a driver, he will usually be willing to do such favors.

Other Transportation Systems

A variety of other services may be used to transport the patient to the day program, including taxis, mass transportation, volunteer drivers, and paid drivers.

Taxis are often much too expensive for the caregiver. Occasionally, a taxi service will establish a special rate and consistent schedule to meet the needs of the patient, and in some states, where Medicaid covers the charges for eligible patients, a taxi will be appropriate and certainly far less expensive than an ambulette service. Overall, however, taxis are most useful as occasional contingency transportation.

Public transportation, such as buses, subways, and trains, are often inappropriate. In addition to requiring that the patient have an escort, their time schedules may not coincide with the arrival and departure times for the program. As patients becomes increasingly impaired, their ability to use this type of transportation is curtailed.

Volunteer drivers are used by some families, through local religious groups or volunteer and service organizations. This should be a private relationship between caregivers and drivers, but the center must keep on file the name, phone number and address of these drivers as you may need to contact them.

Drivers paid by the families are another alternative. The responsibility of locating an individual who wishes to earn extra money by driving and negotiating a fee must remain with the family, and the center staff should not endorse any particular individual as a competent and reliable driver.

Other Problem Areas

Minor difficulties relating to transportation need to be handled before they become major. Depending upon your location and main system of transportation, you may need to solve some of the following problems.

Inclement weather. Develop a policy that gives the center authority to cancel the program or to have a delayed opening when the weather is poor. Although rare, heavy winter storms, flooding, and other significant weather events place a heavy demand on any transportation system. If a major storm is anticipated, it may not be appropriate to have patients brought to the center, when you know from experience that it will be difficult for them to return home.

Even during the worst storms, some caregivers will arrive at the center with their patient. A policy must be developed to allow you to cancel the program when only a few patients arrive.

Be ready to respond to the requests of outside transportation systems, since they may have early pick-ups and change their usual routes during adverse weather conditions. All caregivers should be informed that their relatives may arrive home either early or late.

Patients may experience agitation during transit. As with any agitation problem, try to locate the precursors to it. Does it occur both morning and afternoon? Does the patient have to wait before he can leave? Are families or staff rushing the patient? Some patients become angry when a car or van stops at a red light; others become agitated when another person is dropped off and they must remain in the van.

You may not always be able to locate a source of the problem, especially when the agitation is primarily related to a misinterpretation of events. For example, the patient may see the car or van as the object that separates him from his caregiver or the security of his home. Occasionally, a patient may take a strong dislike to a driver, or become angry when he can no longer drive and must be driven to the program.

Most van systems have rules outlining what is not safe behavior; if a patient regularly removes his seat belt and wanders inside the van, or verbally abuses or physically assaults either the driver or another rider, van transportation is not appropriate.

Some families request that medication be prescribed to ease or reduce anxiety during transit. This decision should only be made in concert with the overall treatment plan for that patient.

Patients who drive themselves to the center can pose special difficulties for the staff. The first issue is whether the program staff feels that the patient is competent to drive, although this may not be an issue in which you choose to become involved. A more important problem that develops when a patient drives himself, either on his own or with someone, is that he inappropriately decides it is time to leave. It is quite difficult to deter an impaired individual, keys in hand, from leaving the center. Whenever possible, therefore, alternatives to a patient's driving himself should be arranged.

Keep current with your transportation system. Once the system is arranged, caregivers and staff members tend to ignore it until problems occur. As with anything that is working well, carefully monitor its operation, since the success of your program depends upon patients' arrival and departure at appropriate times.

Funding, Fees, and Budgets

Any detailed description of obtaining funds for a day care program will quickly become obsolete, and the variability among state laws and among organizational structures is so great that there are no simple solutions to the problem of fundraising. This chapter describes general mechanisms for obtaining funds, and reviews the basic elements of developing a first year budget and patient fee system.

Proprietary Versus Not-for-Profit Organization

Most families and many clinicians are uncomfortable with the concept that organizing and directing a day program is a business, and may also feel that centers which make a profit do so at the expense of quality care. Some programs are developed with a specific goal of making a profit for a corporation and/or for individual investors, but most are organized as voluntary or not-for-profit centers. Whether or not a center has the goal of making a profit, it must oversee billing, general accounting, and the monitoring of cash flow. The fact that a program is not designed for profit must not be confused with a lack of concern that a budget be met and balanced. No program that runs consistently at a loss can continue to provide patient services; it must work to meet its costs, and if possible to exceed them.

A business orientation does not mean poor patient care. Developing and organizing a good quality day care program requires basic business skills, and like any other service program it must pay salaries and related business expenses. Many not-for-profit centers are reviewing and adopting business techniques developed by proprietary organizations, since maximizing the use of funds is universally relevant.

Funding Sources

Most programs receive funds from a variety of government and private sources, which may include "seed money," a specific sum used to help with start-up costs, long-term support such as government funding, and other sources with no restrictions. There are variations among states, but day programs generally receive funding and/or reimbursement from:

- federal, state, and county government agencies, including Medicaid and grants related to aging;
- a variety of private, corporate, or family foundations;
- grants, which may have research, training, or educational components;
- community support groups such as service organizations or auxiliaries;
- private insurance; and
- patient fees.

Key Elements for Program Directors

Obtaining and monitoring funds is frequently the responsibility of the board of directors and chief executive officer, while more routine financial operations are managed by staff. Most day programs assign responsibility for monitoring cash flow and developing new sources of funding to the program director. The task of obtaining funds can interfere significantly with the director's administrative and clinical responsibilities, so time spent on this activity should be carefully monitored, with assistance sought from other staff members, consultants, or board members if appropriate.

Funds will be provided to the program for a specific reason, usually in competition with hundreds of other human service organizations applying for the same health care dollars and foundation support. You will need to provide evidence and facts to any organization to which you apply for reimbursement and/or philanthropic funds, and must effectively communicate how the money will be used. Program directors should always have a fresh supply of project ideas available, so that when financial support becomes available both a track record and new project ideas will be in place.

Many foundation gifts or grants have "strings" attached. Almost every funding source requires periodic reports, which although relatively simple must be done accurately and on time. Occasionally you may apply for and receive a gift or grant from an organization that has either highly specific uses targeted for the funds or unusual reporting requirements; do not apply if you cannot meet these rules. You should also decide if the time invested in applying is justified by the potential results.

Try to avoid having all your funding come from a single source, since funding sources have a way of disappearing when least expected. Although more work is involved, broad-based support from a variety of sources will protect the program.

If you are inexperienced in financial matters, get the help you need. This may involved taking academic course work, or can be as simple as visiting numerous centers and studying their systems. While education provides a good framework, each day center will have a unique system to monitor financial affairs. Both inexperienced directors and those with years of clinical experience but no background in preparing and working with budgets, funding sources, or fee structures, should be given the time and/or financial support to obtain needed training.

Locating Financial Support

Finding avenues of funding can be frustrating, and must be approached systematically. Even when highly organized, overnight changes in laws or rules may leave you with little time to develop and/ or revamp funding proposals. It is far better to delay the opening of a new center than to be faced with curtailing its scope or eliminating it for lack of funds. There are several general strategies for obtaining funding.

Find out what government funding resources are relevant to your program. Planning boards and day program directors should know what government reimbursement and support for which they are qualified, especially what specific funds may be available to programs for the elderly. The difficulty is not in finding these sources, assuming they are available in your state, but in completing a certificate of need, needs assessment, or other application that can take considerable time and energy.

Find out what special or local sources are relevant to your program. You may qualify for certain foundation gifts or grants due to your geographic location, your affiliation with certain organizations, or the types of client you serve. Books are available that detail grant and funding sources. Alternatively, a computer database search may be done on foundation and grant files. This search can be either very general or specialized depending upon the way it is structured. If your local library is unable to provide this service, a reference librarian at a nearby college or university should be able to help.

Local corporations may be interested in providing financial support. Tax relief and positive community relations are frequently the primary reasons for corporate gift giving, but some organizations want to be "good corporate citizens." As discussed above, corporations will be most apt to give money when the results are visible and/or for a specific cause. In return, the day care center should be willing to provide some free training or lecturing for employees of the corporation. For example, most benefit departments would be pleased to schedule a representative of the program for lectures on topics such as "You and Your Aging Parent" or "The Myths and Realities of Alzheimer's Disease."

Be "adopted" by a community service group or auxiliary. Many organizations are skillful in fundraising, and a day program for dementia is an ideal "cause" for fraternal organizations and their auxiliaries, local business groups, college fraternities and sororities, organizations for retired executives, etc. Your goal should be to cultivate their involvement on a permanent basis.

Investigate all options for reimbursement from private insurance. Although rare, some insurance companies will reimburse part or all of a patient's expenses for attending a day care program. Unfortunately, insurance companies consider much of the therapy provided to later stage Alzheimer's patients "maintenance," which is not reimbursable. Very little or no reimbursement can be obtained for activities such as art, music, or dance therapy, therapeutic recreation, or other activity therapies. However, you should be prepared to provide information to insurance carriers when requested to do so by caregivers. Parts of your program that may be reimbursable include speech therapy, occupational therapy, or social work groups.

Most day programs have a flat charge for each day of program attendance. You should be able to provide carriers with a letter written in "insurance bureaucratise" that gives the name and (when applicable) license or registration number of each staff member, their degrees, a brief technical description of the program, and the dates and times the patient attends. This should not be sent to carriers that have already indicated they will not provide reimbursement for any portion of the program.

Consider organizing a yearly fundraising event. Many outside organizations will not provide funds directly to a day care program, but may sponsor or cosponsor a fundraising drive or event with the center. This should go beyond the traditional raffle or yard sale. It should have the backing of a local corporation or business, and you should invite local politicians, celebrities and other notables, with the idea of developing an annual "gala" event which will yield a substantial profit.

Consider hiring a consultant or a part- or full-time grants manager, especially if your program will be largely dependent on grant and foundation support. Grant writing is time consuming and competitive, and many larger centers hire consultants. This can be frustrating for newer, smaller centers that do not have funds for this purpose, in which case the number of grants for which you apply should be limited. Ultimately, the quality rather than the quantity of your applications will determine your level of funding.

Developing a Fee Schedule and Billing Approach

While some programs do not charge for the day care program, most will do so by necessity. It is possible to charge by the hour, or by the service or groups provided, but the simplest method of billing by far is a flat rate for each day that a patient attends the program. If you provide specific billable services, such as certain therapies, supplies, or medications, they can be added to the monthly bill.

Deciding how much to charge is complex. Your rates can be based on costs, both direct and indirect, but must also cover the cost of special or one-time purchases . They should also reflect the current rates for similar services in your area. Before determining a fee structure for your program, you should consider all aspects and ramifications of your decision.

Do not apologize for charging a fee, but do use good community relations techniques when discussing fees with families, the general public, and other agencies, and explain that you provide a highly specialized service. While financial hardship is common in families dealing with Alzheimer's disease, the concept of the day care program must be kept in perspective. An individual may be charged a high fee for a relatively short session of a service such as physical or speech therapy, and it is not unreasonable for a day program that provides six and one-half hours of service to charge an equal or higher amount. Program directors should be prepared to educate potential consumers (see also chapter 14 on community relations).

If you plan to limit admissions to those who pay privately, or who have Medicaid reimbursement, this should be made clear from the beginning. Unless there are alternative services in your community for those who cannot pay, you can expect negative feedback and possibly a loss of referrals and support.

Investigate the option of a sliding fee scale or scholarship programs. Sliding fee scales are usually based on a formula of current income and the number of family members in the household, and should be considered if your center has enough financial support to permit this option. Outside funding sources for both sliding fee scales and scholarship programs are possible if you qualify for foundation funds or for gifts. If you have difficulty in obtaining general purpose funds, it is sometimes easier to obtain funds by campaigning for a scholarship program. It is critical that you be consistent with every applicant, and have a written policy concerning the availability of both sliding scales and scholarship funds.

Developing a Budget

Budgeting and planning are closely interrelated. A budget provides a means of outlining and organizing your priorities and goals as well as a method of internal control. It should allocate all costs of operating the center to specific categories or cost centers, so that it provides useful management information in addition to current information on those sections of the program that are within budget guidelines.

Key Elements in Developing a Budget

Develop a control system so that the staff does not have full independence in spending. While an overly elaborate system is counterproductive, you should require approval for items whose price falls above a set limit, and require written justification for major purchases (capital items). The goal is for spending to coincide with the objectives of the program.

Outline budget categories that reflect major groups of expenses. Each yearly budget must contain the following categories:

- salaries and benefits
- therapy supplies
- food
- medical supplies
- office supplies
- repairs and maintenance
- capital requests
- rent, utilities, and custodial services (some centers may not have this as a distinct cost center)
- transportation

Depending on the finances of your center, the budget may also include:

- travel and education for staff members
- books and periodicals
- outside professional services
- publicity
- professional dues of staff members

Budget control sheets are used to monitor cash flow and as the basis for the succeeding year's budget. How money is spent relative to services provided is core information central to the development of annual statements, grant requests, and promotional materials.

The first year budget will be large due to start-up costs, including furniture, therapy supplies, medical, and safety equipment. Many programs hire consultants or must pay for other professional services (architect, contractor, etc.) during the first year. These and other items must be anticipated and planned for prior to starting the program.

Consider having an emergency fund when beginning a new program. The best of planning committees will make errors in judgment; additionally, changes in rules, codes, and regulations may require significant alterations in your first year budget.

Do not wait to develop other funding sources if the majority of your first year costs are paid by seed money; you cannot assume that funds for continuing the program will be made available without extensive effort.

Other Financial Concerns ⎯⎯⎯⎯⎯⎯⎯⎯⎯⎯⎯⎯⎯⎯

Day program charges and salary ranges for staff members should be consistent with ranges in your area. If you are to attract and keep talented staff members, you need to know what other day programs pay in salaries. Unless you offer services that are unique, your charges must be within the range of those charged by other centers in the area.

A daily charge for the program cannot be set until you have a complete outline of salary, operational, and capital costs for the program.

Be conservative in budgeting money from anticipated patient fees. Many centers are not fully attended in their first year or so of operation. It is better to assume less than full attendance in developing your budget, especially if patient fees will be the primary source of income for the program.

Documentation and Records

Documentation and records must be kept on each patient who attends a day care program. The ultimate responsibility for coordinating program documentation and keeping statistics usually belongs to the program director. The absense of such records equals the absence of information, and without good records it is impossible to review what has been accomplished.

Some centers keep only minimum statistics while others document each activity. The type and style of charting and notekeeping will be dictated by your center's affiliation, licensing, accreditation, and external reporting requirements, as well as by the director's preferred style. Because day care for patients with dementia is not given in an acute care setting, less detailed record keeping is generally required by state agencies and third party payers. Since day care specific to dementia is very new, few if any states have established record and reporting guidelines. Each program director must find out what minimum requirements for clinical record keeping apply to their center. From that minimum, a system can be developed to blend with the program mission, complement staff utilization, and foster optimum patient care.

Purpose of Charting

In addition to providing evidence and data for the center, charting is a useful and practical clinical tool and a tool for planning. A few of the basic intentions of record keeping are:

- charting assists in focusing the staff's attention and their problem solving abilities on the needs of a single patient; this may be the only time that team decisions can be made and agreed upon by the staff;
- the record is permanent and reflects cognitive, physical, and behavioral changes in the patient;
- the chart outlines agreed-upon treatment plans and provides data concerning its progress;
- audits of the charts will provide information needed to satisfy regulatory agencies, third party payers, and other reporting services; and

- charts are a data base that can be used as planning and research tools.

Types of Records _____

Some day centers keep all information relating to a given patient in one record, while others have separate attendance or medication records. The following are typical groupings of information kept in medical model-oriented programs; not all centers are required or should choose to keep this information:

- **admission or fact sheets** with the patient's name, address, care-taker, nearest of kin, names and addresses of children, and date of admission;
- **daily attendance sheets** that record when the patient was present or absent;
- **history and physical health records** provide an initial evaluation of the patient's physical, cognitive, and social status;
- **nurse's medication records** provide an accurate account of the strength or amount of medication, the date and time the medication is given, and the initials of the nurse dispensing the medication;
- **physician's orders sheets** record orders given by the physician with his signature;
- **vital signs sheets** record weight, blood pressure, and possibly pulse and temperature;
- **laboratory reports** contain specific information such as the results of EKG's, laboratory tests, or diagnostic imaging;
- **progress notes** provide an ongoing behavioral account of the patient's progress in the program, and possibly outlining treatment plans and the results of periodic testing;
- **outside records** contain all information gathered on the patient from sources outside the program; and
- **financial and billing records** provide up-to-date financial information and current billing status of the patient.

Minimum Requirements _____

No matter what your program's affiliation or orientation, the following should be considered the **minimum required information;** the director of the program should decide whether it should be kept in one record or as a group of charts.

A list of enrollees and attendance is an absolute necessity. At any given time, the program director should be able to verify the days and dates of attendance of any patient, and great care should be taken to keep this information current and accurate. Data from this record will be useful in:

- monitoring trends in the size of the program;
- planning for possible expansion;
- providing baseline information for current and future budgets;
- verifying attendance for billing disputes; and
- providing information for research, publications, and marketing.

Most centers will want to keep attendance records separate from the main charts, since it is awkward to have an attendance record in twenty or more files. Attandance should be recorded daily, most simply in a chart having a separate sheet for each month, consisting of a grid with the dates across the top and the list of patients on the left side.

A code designating attendance present or absent can be used as long as it is consistent and easy to read, and a daily and monthly attendance total can be kept at the bottom of the sheet. It may also be useful to use this chart for special notes, such as why a program was cancelled on a certain day, a patient's admission and discharge dates, or for designating special billing or financial status by color codings with a highlighter.

A **fact or "face" sheet on each patient** should include the name and address of both the patient and caregiver, a listing of the addresses and telephone numbers of patient's responsible relatives and outside physicians, admissions information such as date of admission or first contact, the referral source, and billing information such as Medicaid identification number, insurance carriers, hospital record number, or charge number.

A **medical information or evaluation form** will be needed for each patient. The depth and sophistication of this material will depend on the type of testing and evaluation services developed and the type of day program and patients admitted to it. It should include:

- a description of the patient's physical and psychosocial status, including both concrete medical information and a descriptive statement of the patient's problems;
- a list of the patient's medications, including name, dosage, and times at which they are to be given;
- special dietary requirements; and

- a list and description of specific problems with daily living or communications skills that would be particularly relevant to the patient's adaptation to a group program.

Progress notes or "charting" for each patient, which may be as simple as a checklist completed on each patient once each month or as complex as individual notes made by a variety of team members every two weeks (see below).

Accident or incidence forms must be used to record any unusual events such as a fall, acute illness, or even a psychiatric emergency. These forms should be kept separately from the main record, since an accident report is a record of internal investigation and is not meant to be shared with outside agencies. The main chart should have a note which outlines the incident in behavioral terms.

Progress Notes

While there are general standards for a good charting system, there are no universal standards for documenting change in individuals who attend adult day programs. Administrators usually agree that the primary reason for having progress notes is to satisfy regulatory agencies, while most clinicians believe that documenting the patient's current status also organizes staff efforts to provide the highest quality patient care.

In designing a system for recording patient progress (or decline), keep in mind that in order to meet these criteria the chart notes must:

- be simple, accurate, legible and containing factual data about the patient rather than staff opinions;
- be signed by the appropriate personnel;
- have some specific relevance to the types of problems with which staff members work; and
- have information from both medical/administrative staff and staff members who provide direct and daily care.

The following suggestions will simplify developing a charting system that will be both simple to use and relevant to the specific needs of your staff.

Team charting, rather than the development of numerous, individual notes completed by different staff members, is most relevant for this patient population. Excessive individual charting wastes staff time that could be better used for patient care, planning, and research. Since day care programs for individuals with dementia is a group effort, patients will receive the best care when all members of the team work with the same information. Team meetings, similar to the "rounds" of the medical community, should be held at regular intervals. If possible, the medical consultant should attend, both because of his perspective on the patients' medical situation and in order to sign orders or write prescriptions based on the information presented. Information from each staff member should be discussed and analyzed to create an accurate and complete picture of each patient's situation. This sharing of observations will also be educational for the staff. A compact behavioral description of the patient's current status and adaptation to the program should be developed, and signed by the director or medical consultant.

Once this system is operational, a large number of charts can be completed in a short amount of time. These meetings should be held in the mornings when the staff is fresh, and they should be separate from team meetings where specific administrative and staffing issues are discussed.

Minimal time intervals between chartings must be established. We have found that the optimal frequency is twice a month. This should be sufficient to satisfy the reporting requirements of most agencies. The minimum interval should be once a month for each patient, since relevant information tends to be forgotten with longer intervals. Weekly chartings are probably excessive, since change is often a slow process in day care programs for patients with Alzheimer's disease, and it is not possible to "document" that patients are improving.

Periodic treatment plans can be incorporated into the team charting, with brief treatment goals outlined for each patient after the observations of the staff are recorded. These short-term plans should be targeted to individual needs. For example, a patient new to the program might have as a treatment goal "assist patient with adaptation to the program and observe for cognitive and behavioral strengths and deficits," while the goal for one who has been in the program for four years might be "assist patient in maintaining appropriate social behavior at lunch by providing verbal cues and hands-on assistance."

These treatment plans should not be complex, as they are not meant to address every problem the patient has. They should focus staff skills on one specific task or problem area. Each team member should be encouraged to contribute both to the development of plans and their execution. Occasionally, a treatment plan will identify one staff member as having primary responsibility, such as the provision of individual therapy for a caregiver by the social worker or specialized nursing care.

After a patient has been in the program for 18 months, it is useful to review all previous treatment plans in the chart. The information in them may be helpful in developing more concrete plans for the patient, while also providing ideas that may assist others.

Most **notes regarding families and caregivers** do not generally need to be recorded separately from the team notes. Information from families should be discussed in the team meeting and integrated into the group note.

Special notes for individual charting may occasionally be needed, as when there is an "incident" which is outside the routine responses or behaviors, a medical emergency, or a crisis for the caregiver. This information may be needed by the administration. The director, social worker, or nurse may be required to write these notes. They should be brief, providing a behavioral account of the situation, evidence that the situation exists, an assessment of the problem, and a suggested course of action. This information can be discussed in the next team conference, and a group note can address the situation.

Testing and Research

Special documentation will be required if your center becomes involved in research or conducts drug treatment trials. Some centers integrate all information from research protocols into the main chart on each patient, while others keep a special research chart that is added to the main chart when the research is completed. Whenever a patient is part of a special research design, a signed consent to participate executed by the patient's closest relative must be placed in the chart. Regardless of the system used, to prevent their loss the main charts should be kept in one place, rather than circulated for the addition of notes.

Special Issues in Documentation

The **right to privacy** of each patient must be protected by the day care staff. Even centers that keep the simplest of records must not release information to other parties without the signed authorization of the patient and/or guardian. Group data that do not identify any person by name or inference can be used without permission.

Personal computers can save considerable time when they are relevant to the recording system and actively used by the staff. Very few facilities have access to a computer during clinical team meetings. A more appropriate role for a computer is to develop a spreadsheet or database tabulation of information that summarizes data for research, professional writing, and planning. If possible, a new program should investigate whether it can have access to a computer. The development of computer-based information is at present missing in most day care centers.

Communication among program directors concerning program documentation and recording needs to be developed. Each center designs a system appropriate to its needs, but better communication and dissemination of information will lessen the need for new programs to develop all new systems. Older programs may learn ways to streamline documentation, ultimately resulting in improved patient care.

Community Relations

A positive rapport with caregivers, community agencies and other service groups does not develop spontaneously. The director of the day care program must disseminate information about it at the local, state, and national levels, and each staff member can and should contribute to this process. This information will identify those who need the service, and provide the information needed for consumers to make full use of it. This chapter reviews key elements needed to develop a good relationship with the community and some basic issues involved in promoting a day care program.

The Promotions Plan

Most day programs for patients with Alzheimer's disease and other dementing illness are developed because people who have experienced dementia in a family member have formed a support group and need a service to provide relief and respite. At the same time, organizations that provide services to elders want to develop and refine services specific to those with dementing illnesses.

Before the day program opens, it must establish its goals and develop a plan for obtaining patients.

Research must be done to estimate the number of people with dementia in your area, and to determine how many primary caregivers are likely to make use of your service. This information can be obtained from a variety of sources, including:

a) local chapters of support groups such as ADRDA, which usually have a mailing list and may allow you to use it;
b) meetings of these groups at which you can contact caregivers directly;
c) county or city offices dealing with aging, which may have local census data on individuals with dementia;
d) county, local, and private social service agencies, which may not be able to provide a list of names but which may have an estimate of numbers; and
e) local geriatric evaluation services, which may range from a single neurologist with special interest in dementia to full scale evaluation programs.

The information gathered through these sources identifies the number of *potential* patients. Some caregivers may want the service, but their family member may be inappropriate for the program; some will have no interest in using the service; and some of the patients may not actually have dementia.

You should also identify existing services in the area. These may include home care services, other day programs, and private practice groups, which may have a vested interest in not sharing information or patients. At this time, the goal is to obtain information, and poor or adversarial relationships with other groups should be avoided.

Develop and deliver a community relations plan, which should formalize the who, where, when, and how of obtaining patients. This involves organizing the information that will be delivered to the community before the program opens, and which will be used to measure its success. A timetable will be needed to evaluate your community relations. Planners should invest time in developing promotions tools—brochures, lectures, radio time, etc.—that are most appropriate for the consumers you want to reach. In many cases a simple program advertisement in a local newspaper or television guide will yield better results than extensive written promotional material. You should focus on those features that make your center and services unique and ways to communicate those features to the general public.

A major mistake frequently made by a new day care center is to believe that it can address all of the needs of patients and caregivers. Providing a few excellent services is better than many primitive or mediocre ones. Reports of poor care will instantly be relayed to other service organizations and to family members.

Internal marketing to educate those who work for or are connected with the day care center is essential to any promotional program. All levels of staff members can contribute strategies that will prove useful.

Evaluate your promotions program, whether it is a sophisticated promotional campaign or a simpler one. Both consumers of the service and referral agencies should be asked at regular intervals for their impressions and suggestions of changes.

Caregivers' responses to the program can be easily determined through interviews and a questionnaire. The director should consider developing a questionnaire that is sent to all caregivers of patients in the program as well as to those who applied but did not choose to participate and those who no longer participate. It should be simple to fill out, delivered with a stamped return envelope, and guaranteed to be kept confidential. The first part should ask for responses to 6-10 statements, using a simple 1-5 rating scale to measure satisfaction, with 1 being extremely unsatisfied and 5 extremely satisfied. The purpose is to identify services that need attention and to highlight those that are well received, not to obtain quantitative evidence. Statements might include:

- The initial explanation of the day care program and its services was adequate and useful.
- The introduction of the patient to the program was well handled.
- Appropriate information is exchanged between staff and family.
- Family support services are useful and adequate.
- The hours of operation of the program are convenient.
- Discharge planning and procedures were handled well by the staff.
- Financial arrangements and billing are accurately managed.

The second part of the questionnaire should consist of open-ended questions that allow families to provide more detailed information, such as:

- What were the greatest benefits of this program for you?
- What were the greatest benefits of the program for your relative who participates in it?
- What were the greatest disadvantages of the program for you and your family?
- What were the greatest disadvantages for your relative who participates?
- If day care had not been available, what alternatives for care would you have most likely pursued?

In addition to querying families, telephone surveys of those agencies that provide referrals to the center will help to pinpoint problems and successes in your referral mechanisms.

Promotional Materials _____

Your program will need to develop promotional materials and continue promoting itself to the public before, during, and after its opening. Your research should allow you to target specific groups and to determine which will benefit from your services. To prevent a lag time between the opening of the center and full registration, community agencies and consumers can be contacted in a variety of ways, including:

- articles in local newspapers, newspaper inserts, and magazines alerting the public to the existence and purpose of the program;

- speaking engagements and the distribution of brochures by the center director at local family service agencies, religious groups, mental health associations, to visiting nurses, etc.; this will alert the professional community to the center's existence and purpose, which may generate referrals;
- enlisting the help of local support groups such as ADRDA to help communicate the mission of the day program to the public; and
- an open house and dedication, which will bring both professionals and families for a tour and an explanation of the program, its physical facilities, and staff.

Public lectures by the center director and staff are one of the best ways to make information about the program available, especially when they involve audiovisual aids such as slides or a videotape. Slides should be made for each component of the program at regular intervals so that your material is always current.

Public Relations

Every day care center will develop an image. All staff members should foster positive public relations and prevent negative or inaccurate perceptions of the program and its goals from developing. Whether staff members are speaking in the community, interviewing caregivers, or giving tours of the facility, they should have facts and evidence at their disposal showing what makes the program unique. Directors must be able to address a variety of issues, including the following.

Day care for patients with dementia is not a "babysitting" service. While you cannot control opinions of the center, you can help to prevent misconceptions about it. Staff members must communicate with outside agencies, groups, and individuals on a professional level, and professional groups should be encouraged to visit the center to observe the types of activities provided.

You cannot meet everyone's needs. A negative public image can develop if a single person communicates serious dissatisfaction. This possibility can be lessened by openly addressing the issue that you cannot help every patient. Concentrate on what you do well, inform the public, and help refer elsewhere those people that you cannot help. At times an individual caregiver will be desperate for "respite," but their relative will be inappropriate for your program. This type of situation and its potential for conflict can seriously disrupt an otherwise solid image. It is important to develop and consistently follow guidelines, rules, and regulations. If your mission is misperceived, people may not consider using your center even though they are appropriate applicants.

If something goes wrong, fix it and move on. Try to develop a reputation for learning from your mistakes, find solutions to your problems, and communicate them to caregivers and professional contacts. Those centers that continue to make the same errors, even after receiving feedback, will lose referrals.

Stress the services that you provide for the patient, in addition to the respite time and support services that you provide for the caregiver. An active community relations program should **emphasize that you are meeting the unique needs of the patient with Alzheimer's disease.**

Avoid feuds with competing services in your area, and concentrate on developing a high standard of care. Day care programs that are secretive about their program plans are usually perceived by other service organizations as dilettantes or agencies trying to hide poor quality care. Try to develop a relationship with other health care providers in your area, and share with others the type of program that you find effective and why you developed your physical space as you did.

Visitors to the Program

Requests to allow visitors and to arrange tours of the program may be frequent, especially as it becomes well known. The positive aspects of giving tours must be balanced against possible negative consequences to staff and/or patients. If dissemination of information is one of your goals, you will need to develop guidelines for visitors.

Visitations must be scheduled by supervising staff, and unscheduled visits should not be permitted. A specific date and time should be arranged, and staff members should know ahead of time who will be visiting.

Visitors, regardless of their backgrounds, should be given instructions before they come into the program area, since interference or inadvertent disruption can occur when outsiders are present. The following rules should be emphasized.

- You are here to *observe*. Do not participate in the group activities unless asked to do so by the group leader.
- Visitors should avoid conversation among themselves, and should not ask questions during program activities, as this can be disruptive to the group.
- Even if you have had experience working with dementia patients,

you cannot understand the complexities of dealing with patients at another center; as a visitor, you are a stranger to the patients.

- Visitors will be given the opportunity to meet with a member of the staff before leaving to discuss any questions that may arise.
- If the patients are unusually agitated, the visit may have to be curtailed or rescheduled. Patient safety will always be the first priority. If a staff member asks you to leave the patient area, do so and return to the director's office.

Limit the number of visitors on any given day. The presence of more than two or three extra people can be draining for the staff. If a large group wishes to visit, and you have sufficient staff, they should be divided into groups of two or three.

Have an occasional moratorium on visitors to ease the strain on the staff. You should also avoid having visitors during holidays, vacation times, or times when you are short-staffed.

Monitor the time spent with visitors, which can become time-consuming, especially if your center is well known. Additionally, you should have clearly defined limits concerning how much information you will provide, and how much training and consultation you will do. Some individuals may try to use your expertise inappropriately, repackage it and "sell" it back into the community.

Training and Consulting

Staff members may be asked to plan and lead seminars, provide direct training to staff at other programs, or to do consulting work. Your policies on this topic should be communicated to all program staff, and should include the following.

The development of a private practice is encouraged by some centers, while others forbid staff members to work privately with program patients or their relatives. This issue should be clearly addressed and guidelines provided.

The center should encourage staff members to be involved in education and training programs. Public speaking and writing helps to develop a good rapport with outside agencies, as well as being one of the best boosts to any career. Your staff members should be encouraged to present material on your program to both professional and lay groups. If staff members are not comfortable with public speaking, they should be encouraged to write for professional publications. Your staff members' increased visibility in their own areas of professional expertise is good public relations for your program as well as valuable for the individuals themselves.

Rules regarding the acceptance of honoraria must be developed. Many organizations provide honoraria for speakers in addition to travel and expenses. Some programs allow staff members to keep honoraria received for speaking engagements, while others require that they be donated to the program. Whatever policy you adopt, it should be consistent for staff members throughout the center, and not dependent on length of tenure or level within the organization.

The Media

Most day centers will at some time be asked if they can be featured in newspaper or magazine articles, or in radio or television programs. There is a potential for both positive and negative community relations in participating in such media events. The center director must carefully structure such activities, and address the following issues.

Obtain releases from patients and/or families if patients will be on film, referred to in print, or their names used in any way. This should involve receiving a *signed* response to a letter of explanation sent to the family. It is not unusual for a media representative to give very little notice, which can be disruptive in terms of staff time and energy.

Patients whose families do not wish them to be photographed should probably remain home on a day when a television group is visiting, as it is often impossible to run two separate groups on a day when staff members are involved with the media.

Find out the overall purpose of the group that is filming or writing about the program. Identify whether the staff, patients, or caregivers will be the main focus of the story, and request information on the length of the article or film, where and when it will be used, etc. It is not uncommon for a film crew to want to spend extensive time at your center but to plan to use it as background material, or for a piece emphasizing a topic other than day care programs for patients with dementia. This information should be made available beforehand and in writing.

Do not hesitate to give directions to producers, directors, and photographers. The safety and security of the program is your first priority, and visitors from the media must take cues and suggestions from staff. They often welcome suggestions concerning which patients they should emphasize, what activities would best describe the program, and how to be least disruptive.

If possible, see the product before the general public does. You should offer your assistance, since most writers and producers are not experts in the field of dementia and their interpretation of events in your program may not be correct.

Overall, any public relations event, from the development of a program logo and brochure to an open house or "gala" event, will require a tremendous amount of work. The end result will, more often than not, far outweigh the aggravation and time involved. Your focus should always be on refining the program and its services.

Subject Index